W

Patient Safety

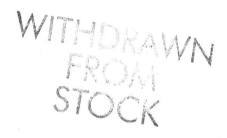

Patient Safety

An Essential Guide

Heather Gluyas
Paul Morrison

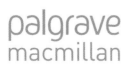

palgrave
macmillan

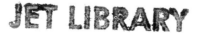

First published 2013 by
PALGRAVE MACMILLAN

Palgrave Macmillan in the UK is an imprint of Macmillan Publishers
Limited, registered in England, company number 785998, of Houndmills,
Basingstoke, Hampshire RG21 6XS.

Palgrave Macmillan in the US is a division of St Martin's Press LLC,
175 Fifth Avenue, New York, NY 10010.

Palgrave Macmillan is the global academic imprint of the above companies
and has companies and representatives throughout the world.

Palgrave® and Macmillan® are registered trademarks in the United States,
the United Kingdom, Europe and other countries

ISBN: 978-0-230-35496-8 paperback

This book is printed on paper suitable for recycling and made from fully
managed and sustained forest sources. Logging, pulping and manufacturing
processes are expected to conform to the environmental regulations of the
country of origin.

A catalogue record for this book is available from the British Library.

A catalog record for this book is available from the Library of Congress.

Typeset by Cambrian Typesetters, Camberley, Surrey

Printed in China

Dedicated to Alan, Franziska, Sarah and Maeve

Contents

Figures

Tables

Acknowledgements

The authors would like to acknowledge our colleagues Michelle Bradshaw, Susanne Aitken, Peter Wall and Sarah Smith who shared their knowledge and experiences with us and helped shape our book to make it meaningful to all clinicians in the pursuit of patient safety. The authors and publishers also wish to thank BMJ Publishing Group Ltd for permission to reproduce Figure 1.1 Swiss Cheese model by J. Reason, originally from *Human error: Models and management* in British Medical Journal v320 © 2000 and Figure 7.2 Three bucket self-assessment tool by J. Reason, originally from *Beyond the Organisational Accident* in Quality and Safety in Healthcare v13 suppl 2 © 2004; World Health Organization for the Letter from Alice in Exercise 2.3, originally from *WHO Patient Safety Curriculum Guide for Medical Schools* (available at whqlibdoc.who.int/publications/2009/9789241598316_eng.pdf) © 2009, and we also acknowledge the *WHO Patient Safety Curriculum Guide* (2011) and its role in this book; the Agency for Healthcare Research and Quality for case studies in Chapters 4, 5, 6 and 7 found within *Cases and Commentaries* available through www.webmm.ahrq.gov/cases.aspx; Australian Commission on Safety and Quality in Healthcare for Table 4.1 Good practice principles when prescribing medication, originally from *Recommendations for Terminology, Abbreviations and Symbols used in the Prescribing and Administration of Medicines* © 2010, and W.W. Norton and Company, Inc for Figure 4.2 What is this? by V. Ramachandran, originally Fig 2.8 (a pig rump), from *The Tell-tale Brain: A neuroscientists quest for what makes us human*. Copyright © 2011.

Introduction

This is a book about patient safety. It is not intended as an academic text but rather a practical guide for health practitioners to heighten personal awareness of safety issues and harness their commitment to patient safety. It does so by providing current information about patient safety and strategies which practitioners, as individuals, can implement in their practice and their workplace. While not claiming to be an academic text the content is informed by current research and literature about the problems and challenges faced by practitioners when trying to achieve the goal of patient safety.

The authors have a combined experience covering both the academic setting (undergraduate and postgraduate health students) and a variety of clinical settings with a focus on clinical governance and patient safety. This experience – backed up by findings reported in the literature [1] – has provided ample evidence that, while there is an abundance of research and literature about patient safety, this area often is not prioritised in the context of everyday healthcare delivery. This is not because there is a lack of genuine commitment to patient care, patient safety and maximising positive outcomes for patients, but because it can become lost in the day-to-day work pressures and resource and time constraints typical of modern health systems. A commitment to patient safety may be further weakened by increasing patient acuity, the use of more complex technology and changing patient expectations [2].

This book has arisen out of frustration that caring and dedicated health professionals involved in all aspects of healthcare are unable to overcome the barriers to improving patient safety statistics. It is hoped that its format – presenting research and principles about patient safety intertwined with realistic case studies – will help the reader to relate the theory to everyday practice. Reflective exercises/activities are included so that readers can develop a deeper understanding of the concepts presented, especially as they apply within the context of their own practice.

The aims of this book then are threefold. It aims, firstly, to familiarise student health practitioners with the concept of patient safety, and secondly, to help health practitioners (both new and more experienced) who are searching for ways to put the concept of patient safety into practice in their everyday clinical context. Finally, this book is for those managers and administrators who are familiar with the theories and concepts related to the promotion of patient safety but are seeking to understand the clinical perspective.

Is there really a need for a book like this? Why can't medical and nursing staff be relied on to provide the best possible care and make sure that errors in care do not happen? Surely the chances that patients will suffer an adverse event arising from an error are very low? These are all fair questions, but the answer to them is 'No'. The chances of a patient experiencing an adverse event are much higher than those when partaking in some sports that most would consider far more dangerous. For instance, the mortality rate for hang-gliding, scuba diving, parachuting or mountaineering has been calculated as between 0.59 and 0.0029 per hundred participants [3]. Compare this with the statistics for patients in hospitals: Studies have identified that 1 in 10 patients will experience an adverse event as a result of an error in their care [4]. Of the 1 in 10 patients who suffer an adverse event:

- 1 in 5 will suffer severe injury
- 1 in 30 will die as a result of the adverse event [5–7].

The research literature tells us that between 50 and 80 per cent of these adverse events are preventable. However, very few of them are due to negligence. Their financial cost is astronomical and their human cost incalculable for all those involved [6, 8, 9]. These statistics demonstrate there is definitely a challenge in being able to assure patients they are safe in hospital. The notion of safety cannot be taken as a 'given' as far as patients, families and professions are concerned.

For as long as patients have been receiving care from health professionals, it is likely that errors and adverse events have occurred. However, in the main, these were not identified or discussed and were thought to be very rare. If they came to the notice of patients or other health professionals the assumption was that the error or adverse event occurred because the health professional was sloppy, unsafe, careless, inattentive or negligent [10]. The focus was on blaming the individual who committed the error, with the solution being to remediate the poor behaviour or dismiss them from the organisation [10–12].

The challenge of improving patient safety is not limited to a single health system. There have been different reports and studies across many countries. In 2000 in the United States (US) the Institute of

Medicine (IOM) published the report *To Err is Human* [13]. This report brought together research findings showing that between 44,000 and 98,000 patients in the US were injured each year by adverse events while hospitalised. To make these figures more meaningful the report demonstrated that more patients died from an adverse event than died from either motor vehicle accidents, breast cancer or AIDS. Pivotally, the report emphasised that although individuals at the point of care made the errors, the *problem lay within the systems* they worked in, which made it more likely errors would occur. So the focus shifted from 'bad people' to 'poor systems'.

In the United Kingdom (UK) the high profile investigation into poor outcomes for paediatric cardiac surgery at the Royal Bristol Infirmary alerted the public to the issue of inadequate care and patient safety [14, 15]. In the shadow of this investigation, but prior to the release of the final report of the Bristol Inquiry team, the UK Government released a report of an expert group, led by Dr Liam Donaldson, Chief Medical Officer, called *An Organisation with a Memory* [16]. This report also highlighted the need to look at the reasons errors occurred, rather than blaming the individuals involved. The report acknowledged that there had been little systematic learning from patient safety incidents and service failure in the National Health Service in the past, and drew attention to the scale of the problem of potentially avoidable events that result in unintended harm to patients.

In Australia a study by Wilson et al. [17] estimated 18,000 deaths and 17,000 permanent disabilities occur each year to patients in Australian hospitals as a result of preventable errors. These findings led to the Australian Commonwealth and State Health Ministers establishing the Australian Council for Safety and Quality in Health Care (ACSQHC; now called the Australian Commission for Safety and Quality in Healthcare).

These reports, as well as studies in other developed countries including Denmark, New Zealand, Canada and France, demonstrated that there was a very significant problem with errors and adverse events, beyond these being an occasional occurrence [7]. They also identified that if improvement was to be achieved then attention had to be diverted away from blaming people. Instead, there needed to be a focus on understanding why errors occurred.

While the focus of this book is on developed countries it is important to recognise that the challenge of improving patient safety is not limited to them. A recent study of 26 hospitals in transitional and developing countries concluded there was a significant problem regarding patient safety and adverse events. In reviewing 15,548 patient records this study identified that 8.2 per cent showed at least one adverse event, with 30 per cent associated with the death of the patient. Of the adverse events identified, 83 per cent were judged as preventable [18]. Supporting these findings, the World Health Organization (WHO) has identified that the risk of an adverse event is much higher in such countries than in developed ones, citing that the risk of a patient acquiring a healthcare related infection is 20 times higher [19].

This awareness about the risks to patient safety has begun to form a major focus for health service providers, the governments that manage and regulate the provision of health services, and the communities and consumers (patients and families) who are recipients of the care. Governments have committed resources to build capacity within organisations that supports patient safety and quality, and there has been a growth in research into areas that contribute to patient safety [20]. Most healthcare organisations have adopted systems and processes that support safe care. However, studies still identify a deficit of knowledge about the issues around patient safety within the health professional workforce [1]. The World Health Organization has recognised that there are a number of impediments to improving patient safety education, and to address these has developed a *Patient Safety Curriculum* for use internationally in the higher education sector [1]. The WHO guide identifies 11 topics that are considered essential to inform patient safety knowledge in health practitioners. Our book is informed by a selection of these topics, as illustrated in Table 0.1. A summary of the themes of each chapter as related to the WHO curriculum topics is also provided at the end of each chapter.

There are two areas of patient safety we have not been able to cover in this book: pressure areas and falls. These have been omitted due to space constraints, not because of their lack of importance. The occurrence of falls and pressure areas within acute hospitals and the community setting is high. The falls incident rate is between 1.9 and 3 per cent of all hospitalisations, and the prevalence rate of pressure ulcers is between 4 and 27 per cent [1, 21–23]. There has been an enormous amount of research into identifying profiles of patients at particular risk of falls and pressure ulcers. As well, there are many evidence based care protocols that lessen the likelihood of falls, pressure ulcers and healthcare acquired infections [1, 24, 25]. However, there is mounting evidence that the risk assessment tools and prevention strategies for these types of incidents are not being universally applied [26]. The simplicity of interventions versus the cost saving in dollars and in

Table 0.1   The WHO curriculum topics linked to chapters

WHO curriculum topic*	Patient Safety: An Essential Guide
What is patient safety?	Chapter 1
Why human factors are important for patient safety	Chapters 1, 3, 4, 5, 6, 7, 8
Understanding systems and the complexity of care	Chapter 1
Being an effective team player	Chapters 5, 7
Learning from errors to prevent harm	Chapter 6
Understanding and managing clinical risk	Chapter 6
Using quality improvement methods to improve care	Chapter 8
Engaging with patients and carers	Chapter 2
Infection prevention and control	Chapter 3
Patient safety and invasive procedures	Indirectly covered in Chapters 1, 2, 3, 5, 7, 8
Improving medication safety	Chapter 4

*WHO Patient Safety Curriculum Guide: Multi-professional edition (2011) [1: 18–19].

human impact seems not to attract the excitement and attention that would focus the resources and support required to achieve the major changes which would improve outcomes for patients. Until this happens there will be little impact on the incidence rates of falls and pressure areas. Falls and pressure areas are a significant patient safety issue, and individual healthcare practitioners have a key part to play in their prevention. The key messages for health practitioners to minimise risk of falls and pressure areas are:

- ensure all patients are risk-screened on admission
- institute active prevention strategies to minimise the risks identified in the assessment
- take the opportunity to educate patients and families of the risks and minimisation strategies
- ensure that they remain abreast of current research about falls and pressure areas.

The book is presented in a format that allows you to skip back and forth depending on what is relevant for you, or it can be read straight through. Take time to do the exercises – they will help you to incorporate the information presented into your practice. At the end of each chapter the Exercise Feedback section provides an overview of the key points of the chapter.

Chapter 1 sets the scene by introducing the background of the patient safety movement. The research literature is explored to appreciate the different perspectives used to understand the cognitive processes involved, and the organisational factors that increase the likelihood that humans will make errors. Finally, the discipline of human factors is introduced as a platform for further discussion throughout the book to identify strategies in error prone situations that may avert errors.

Chapter 2 explores patient safety from the patients' perspective, especially in terms of the management and prevention of errors. The topics discussed include how to communicate with patients and families to explain risk and manage adverse events. In addition, opportunities to partner with patients to prevent errors are identified.

Chapter 3 looks at the common area of risk for all patients who are receiving acute care. The occurrence of healthcare acquired infections within acute hospitals is high – so much so that health professionals can become desensitised to the frequency of these events. There are many evidence based care protocols that lessen the likelihood of healthcare acquired infections. These will be reviewed so that health practitioners can both implement and champion them within their own care contexts.

Chapter 4 looks at the elements of the medication administration system and the types of errors that occur at each stage of the process, including prescription, dispensing and administration. Improving medication safety is paramount as medication errors are one of the most common adverse events. Medication errors are discussed with reference to our knowledge of human factors. Finally, strategies that individual health practitioners can use to minimise the potential for errors are examined.

Chapter 5 explores the critical role of communication within a team to achieving optimal patient safety. The barriers to effective team communication are discussed, including interpersonal relationships and attitudes, group and peer pressure, and hierarchical structure of healthcare teams that lead to an authority gradient. Strategies to improve communication effectiveness such as the SBAR and CUSP tool are presented. There is a focus on the key areas in which these tools can be utilised for better outcomes, including the scenarios of the deteriorating patient, handover and patient handoffs.

Chapter 6 reviews the common organisational adverse incident reporting systems. The value of adverse event/incident reporting systems is in allowing analysis of the reports to identify factors that led to incidents and then the development of strategies to prevent or minimise the errors. Quality management and risk management are discussed as organisational responses to reduce errors. The role of the individual health practitioner in the reporting and analysis of incidents is then explored.

Chapter 7 explores the human side of safe work practices by considering some of the psychological processes that can influence safety: self-awareness, values and commitment to safe work practices. These can be enhanced as individual health practitioners develop situational awareness and improve communication in their everyday practice and in emergency/crisis situations.

Chapter 8 looks at the goals for the future of patient safety and the role of individual health practitioners in championing the lessons learnt so far. There is a brief discussion about the principles of change management and how individuals can implement patient safety principles in their workplace. Finally, a list of resources that are available for learning more about patient safety concepts is presented.

We hope that this book provides you with the skills and knowledge to bridge the gap between theory and practice, and as a result that patients' risk of an adverse event while they are receiving care is diminished.

References

1. *WHO Patient Safety Curriculum Guide: Multi-professional edition*, 2011, Geneva: World Health Organization.
2. Saint, S., et al., *Introducing the patient safety professional.* Journal of Patient Safety, 2011. **7**(4): 175–180.
3. Windsor, J., et al., *Mountain mortality: A review of deaths that occur during recreational activities in the mountains.* Postgraduate Medical Journal, 2009. **85**: 316–321.
4. O'Leary, D. and L. Leape, *Teaching physicians to provide safe patient care*, in *Patient Safety Handbook*, B. Youngberg, ed. 2013, Maryland: James & Bartlett Learning.
5. Carayon, P., ed. *Handbook of Human Factors and Ergonomics in Health Care and Patient Safety*. 2nd ed. *Human Factors and Ergonomics*, G. Salvendy, ed. 2012, Boca Raton, Florida: CRC Press.
6. de Vries, E., et al., *The incidence and nature of in-hospital adverse events: A systematic review.* Quality and Safety in Health Care, 2007. **17**(3): 216–223.
7. Reynard, J., J. Reynolds, and P. Stevenson, *Practical Patient Safety*, 2009, Oxford: Oxford University Press.
8. McGlynn, E., et al., *The quality of health care delivered to adults in the United States.* New England Journal of Medicine, 2003. **348**: 2635–2645.

9.   Runciman, B., et al., *CareTrack: Assessing the appropriateness of health care delivery in Australia*. MJA, 2012. **197**(2): 100–105.

10. Runciman, W., A. Merry, and M. Walton, *Safety and Ethics in Healthcare: A guide to getting it right*, 2007, Aldershot, Hampshire: Ashgate Publishing.

11. Parker, D. and R. Lawton, *Psychological approaches to patient safety*, in *Patient Safety: Research into practice*, K. Walshe and R. Boaden, eds. 2006, Maidenhead, Berkshire: Open University Press: 31–40.

12. Carroll, J. and M. Quijada, *Redirecting traditional professional values to support safety: Changing organisational culture in health care*. Quality and Safety in Health Care, 2004. **13**: 16–21.

13. IOM, *To Err is Human: Building a safer health care system*, 2000, Washington, DC: National Academy Press.

14. Walshe, K. and N. Offen, *A very public failure: Lessons for quality improvement in healthcare organisations from the Bristol Royal Infirmary*. Quality and Safety in Health Care, 2001. **10**: 250–256.

15. Hindle, D., et al., *Patient Safety: A comparative analysis of eight inquiries in six countries*, 2006, Sydney: Centre for Clinical Governance, University of New South Wales.

16. *An Organisation with a Memory: Report of an expert group on learning from adverse events in the National Health Service*, 2000, London: Department of Health.

17. Wilson, R., et al., *The quality in Australian health care study*. MJA, 1995. **193**: 458–471.

18. Wilson, R., et al., *Patient safety in developing countries: Retrospective estimation of scale and nature of harm to patients in hospital*. BMJ, 2012. **344**: e832.

19. *Patients for Patient Safety – Statement of case*, Geneva: World Health Organization.

20. Wolff, A. and S. Taylor, *Enhancing Patient Safety: A practical guide to improving quality and safety in hospitals*, 2009, Sydney: MJA Books.

21. Suurmond, J., *Explaining ethnic disparities in patient safety: A qualitative analysis*. American Journal of Public Health, 2010. **100**(Suppl. 1): S113–117.

22. Walshe, K., *Pseudoinnovation: The development and spread of healthcare quality improvement methodologies*. International Journal for Quality in Health Care, 2009. **21**(3): 153–159.

23. Paterson, I. and I. Burns, *Making practice perfect*. Nursing Management – UK, 2007. **14**(1): 12–16.

24. Parker, L., et al., *Creating quality improvement dialogue utilizing knowledge from frontline staff, managers and experts to foster health care quality improvement*. Quality Health Research, 2009. **19**(1): 229–242.

25. Henderson, S., *Power imbalance between nurses and patients: A potential inhibitor of partnership in care*. Journal of Clinical Nursing, 2003. **12**: 501–508.

26. Manser, T., et al., *Team communication during patient handover from the operating room: More than facts and figures*. Human Factors, 2013. **55**(1): 136–156.

1

What Do We Mean By Patient Safety?

Introduction

> It may seem a strange principle to enunciate as the very first require-
> ment in a Hospital that it should do the sick no harm. (Florence
> Nightingale, 1859)

Patients come in all shapes and sizes with many different types of
illnesses and conditions. Their backgrounds can range from very poor
to very wealthy, from educated to illiterate and from any range of
cultural environments. But no matter the background or patient condition our role as health professionals is to ensure that while we are part
of their care team the care they receive is of the highest quality possible. Unfortunately, in many cases our patients experience adverse
events during their care that are not a result of their illness but rather a
result of something we as health professionals have or have not done.
It might be that the wrong medication was given to a patient or maybe
that a medication was completely forgotten. It could be that the hand
washing routine before attending to a patient was overlooked, or it
might be that the wrong procedure was carried out on a patient. But
whatever the error, you can be fairly certain that the health professional
involved did not intentionally make an error. So why do errors happen?
And what can we do to prevent them?

In the Introduction we noted that 10 per cent of patients experience
an adverse event, and that 1 in 5 of these will suffer a serious injury from
the adverse event – and 1 in 30 of these will die as a result [1–4]. Knowing
the incidence of adverse events leads to many questions, such as: why do
errors happen, and what can we as individual health professional and
healthcare organisations do to prevent them? In this chapter we will
explore some of the explanations provided in the research literature for

9

why errors happen. However, before we start it is important to define the terminology that we will be using regarding the terms 'error' and 'adverse event'. These terms are fundamental to any discussion on patient safety but their interpretation can vary between practitioners. The definitions we will use in this book are those agreed by WHO [5] for usage in discussions and research about patient safety.

Definitions

In the context of patient safety an *error* is an occurrence that happens because of:

- failure to do something that should have been done to or for a patient (error of omission)
- doing the wrong thing to or for a patient (error of commission) [5].

An example in the clinical context is a situation where a diabetic patient did not receive the insulin charted for a particular time – this is an *error* (of omission) because something was not done for the patient when it should have been. However, if the patient received insulin at the scheduled time but it was the wrong dose of insulin this is still an *error* (of commission) because the wrong thing was done for the patient.

When we use the term *adverse event* we are describing injury or harm that occurs to a patient as a result of the healthcare they received rather than from their underlying medical condition. Not all *adverse events* are the result of *errors* [5]. Consider the following situation: A diabetic patient who has a severe infection suffers several hyperglycaemic episodes (raised blood glucose) secondary to the increased metabolic demands of the infective process – this *adverse event* for the patient is not the result of an *error*. Another diabetic patient suffers a severe hyperglycaemic episode as a result of the morning dose of insulin not being given by the assigned nurse at the scheduled time – this is an *adverse event* as a result of an *error*.

Of course, sometimes an error occurs and due to good fortune does not lead to an adverse event for the patient. This is termed a *near miss*. An example of this is when a medication is charted incorrectly for a patient but it is recognised by the nurse who intervenes and ensures the medication is charted correctly. These types of errors are problematic as they are mostly not reported and so we lose the opportunity to learn from them and put processes in place to prevent the same thing happening again [6]. We will be talking about this in more detail in Chapter 6.

Other terminology that you will encounter includes a care process that is described as occurring at the *sharp end*, which refers to the care delivered at the point of care – for instance the nurse doing the dressing or the doctor prescribing the medication. The *blunt end*, on the other hand, refers to those parts of the care process that are removed from the direct point of care but influence the care delivered. Examples of those at the *blunt end* are managers, administrators, accreditors and policy makers. Errors that occur at the *sharp end* of care are described as *active errors* and those that occur at the *blunt end* are described as *latent errors* [7]. Consider the scenario of a nurse confusing the required dosage of medication and administering morphine 25 mg instead of 2.5 mg. This is an *active error* and might have the contributing factors of stress, fatigue, noisy work environment, or multiple interruptions which may have distracted the nurse and led to her calculating the dose incorrectly. The *latent errors* that may have contributed to this active error might be the decision by the ward designer to place the drug cupboard where there is poor lighting, or the administrator deciding to decrease the funding for staff so a newly qualified graduate nurse is working unsupported, or the decision by the pharmacist to stock only one concentration of morphine so the nurse is having to work out the dosage. We will explore these concepts further later in this chapter.

In the next section we will review several different research perspectives that provide some understanding of why errors occur. But firstly, we suggest you complete the following exercise and then compare your findings with the Exercise Feedback at the end of the chapter.

Exercise 1.1

Aim of the exercise: To explore different perspectives on understanding why errors occur.

What to do:

1. Identify a specific minor error you have made or observed recently. Preferably the error will be one that has happened in the clinical area – for example, a late or missed medication, missed or late routine observations, treatment for abnormal test results not being actioned in a timely manner, or a particular aspect of a patient's treatment requirements not being handed over at the change of shift. If you can't think of a clinical error then reflect on

other 'everyday errors' that you may have made recently – for example, forgetting to buy something you needed at home, missing a train, not indicating when changing traffic lanes or not being able to recall where you put the car keys.

2. Write down what happened, and then write a list of factors that contributed to the error. When you are doing this think about what was happening around you, what was happening in your life at the time and what other things you had to do before, after and at the same time. In particular see if you can recall and label any emotions that were prevalent. Also, note down any other factors that you think may have contributed to the error happening at that particular time.

3. Discuss your notes with colleagues (or friends) and see if you can note any common reasons you have all identified that contribute to how errors occur. Add to your own list any contributing factors that others have identified which may have contributed to your error.

4. Which items on the list grab your attention? What do these suggest to you that might be useful in your own work setting? Note these down also.

5. Keep this list, as you will need it in the next exercise.

6. Compare your findings with the Exercise Feedback section at the end of the chapter.

Why Do Errors Happen?

Health professionals are well educated and committed to giving high quality care to patients. When an error occurs the reasons are rarely because the person who made the error is incompetent. Rather, there are many contributing factors when an error occurs. Some of these factors are related to the way we as humans think and act when we are carrying out tasks (human cognition) and some are related to the complex systems that operate within healthcare organisations [8, 9].

Errors can be classified in several different ways. For instance, they may be classified according to cognitive stage that they occur – that is, at the planning stage (mistakes), storage stage (lapses) or execution stage (slips). They may also be classified as knowledge based (error in conscious analysis of stored knowledge), skill based (error in retrieving or executing stored knowledge), rule based (error when carrying out a familiar task without conscious thought) or, as previously noted, as errors of commission or omission [10].

Cognition and errors

For the purpose of this discussion about errors and the effect of cognition, we are referring to how we acquire knowledge and understanding from what is going on around us, reviewing past experiences, and then applying this to decisions, tasks and reasoning in a given situation [3, 7, 11]. These cognition processes can be affected by environmental, emotional or physical distractions – for example, maybe the workplace is very busy and lots of people are trying to get our attention at once; or maybe we are worried about how we can pay all our bills; or maybe we are sick or hung-over from too much alcohol the night before.

There are two vital areas of focus when we look at cognition in relation to errors. These are deliberate conscious actions and automatic behaviour. When we are doing something that is new or requires our attention we pay conscious attention to how we do it. This tends to be in the situation where the task is new or complicated. An example would be when we are learning to drive for the first time or when we use a new piece of machinery or a new software program. However, many of the tasks we undertake we do automatically with very little conscious thought, such as when we are driving on a routine journey home from work or hanging the washing on the line. This automatic behaviour allows us to multi-task [12]. There are three types of errors associated with these cognitive states: mistakes, lapses and slips [13].

Some mistakes are associated with conscious thought. When we are consciously undertaking an action we use 'stored' solutions. These can be based on our knowledge of similar situations or actions. However, to do this we must make an assessment of the situation and then choose the appropriate action. Moreover, when we are assessing a situation our bias is to use solutions that have worked before, pattern matching to similar situations, or to use the first solution we think of and then discount any evidence that does not support the initial assessment [12]. These biases are actually very handy and in many cases work well, but the more complicated or novel the situation the more likely we are to make an incorrect assessment and therefore choose the wrong action. Here is an example. In one particular ward there were multiple occasions when the emergency bell had been initiated in the patients' rooms but over the last year it had never been an emergency – rather it was because patients had tended to push the emergency call bell instead of the patient assist bell. So, when the ward is busy the nurses do not respond immediately to emergency call bells in the patient rooms until one day it is an emergency and because no one responds immediately appropriate care is delayed. Mistakes, then, are when we complete the action successfully but it is the wrong action for the situation [7, 11]. Mistakes also fit into the category of knowledge and rule based errors as they are related to how we retrieve and process information to make decisions [14].

Slips and lapses are both associated with automatic behaviour when our attention is diverted elsewhere. Lapses are where we intend to do something but forget to carry it out; for instance we may have been asked to get a drink for the patient but on our way to get it the phone goes so we answer that and deal with the call and then forget completely about the drink. Slips are where we undertake a task without conscious thought and in doing this we don't quite get all the actions required to do the task in the right order or we leave one of the actions out – for instance when we pour the hot water from the kettle into the cup forgetting to put in the teabag! This can happen because our attention is diverted elsewhere while we are doing the task (maybe daydreaming!) or we are doing several things at the same time. So slips and lapses are when we take the right action but do it incorrectly [7, 11]. Slips and lapses fit into the category of skill based errors.

Having discussed the unintentional slips, lapses and mistakes there is a further type of error that occurs when an action deviates from the rules. These are called violations, and happen when the person undertaking an action *intentionally* deviates from the rules, protocols, policies, and so on. There may be several reasons for the person making a conscious decision to do this. Firstly, they may feel the rules don't apply to their situation, maybe because they have the skill and knowledge that allows them to discount the rules. An example of this would be the requirement to wear personal protection like gloves and glasses when changing urinary catheter bags but the person decides not to do this because the technique they use minimises the chances of splashes and therefore they don't think it is necessary [3].

The second type of violation arises because the resources required are not available or it is difficult or impossible to apply the rule in the particular situation. An example of this would be the requirement to wash hands between different patient encounters but there are no hand basins or no hand gel located close to patient care areas [3].

While violations involve conscious intention to deviate from rules, errors and subsequent adverse events that occur as a result of these are not intended. This distinction is important as it differentiates violations from the very rare event where harm is caused by the action of a health professional who undertakes the action consciously with the intention of deliberately harming a patient [15].

The solution to preventing slips, lapses, mistakes and violations does not lie with blaming the person. Instead we must recognise that humans are fallible as a result of the way we function cognitively. The likelihood of mistakes, slips and lapses increases if we are stressed, distracted, tired or unwell. What we must recognise is that slips and lapses present a huge risk to patients as so much of what is done in healthcare is done automatically. In addition, mistakes and violations also pose a risk to patients as the technological and fast paced healthcare environment requires complex decisions to be made where resources and support may be lacking. Telling someone that they must do better or pay attention is not always going to solve the problem – so other solutions must be identified.

Having examined the influence of human cognition on errors we will now look at the complex systems that make up any healthcare organisation and then discuss how this complexity can influence the likelihood of an error occurring by increasing stress or distraction.

Complex systems

Healthcare organisations cover a vast array of differing care provision and many different institutions of varying size and capacity. The organisations may be housed in a single building, or across several campuses and sites. The care may be specialised tertiary care, secondary care or primary care. The patients may have a short episode of care or have ongoing complex acute or chronic healthcare needs. However, no matter the type or size of organisation, there will be many complex and interacting systems that cooperate to provide care. These systems include the increasing fragmentation of care across multiple departments and processes that make up any organisation, as well as growing specialisation of health professionals, and the health professional culture within healthcare organisations. Complexity increases the risks within a system.

Multiple departments and processes

There are many different departments and types of systems and processes across a healthcare organisation. These might include: medical records; human resources; many clinical departments, for example physiotherapy, pharmacy, radiology, operating theatre; numerous wards such as medical, surgical, paediatrics; biomedical engineering; building maintenance; and catering. All are required to work together to different degrees to deliver high quality care and treatment to patients and their families. Within each of these departments there are interconnected systems and processes, which leads to even further complexity. For instance, if we look at operating theatres, there may be anaesthetics, speciality theatres, sterilising department, recovery room and many others.

Increasing specialisation

As healthcare has become more technical and complex there has been an increase in specialisation in all health professions. This specialisation has led to considerable improvements in care, with improved diagnosis and treatments. But there has been a downside in that it makes errors of care more likely to occur [16].

If we look at nursing as an example, there was a time when a nurse provided many different aspects of care to patients including interventions that are now the domain of other professions such as physiotherapists, occupational therapists, dieticians, respiratory therapists and phlebotomists. As well, many tasks now considered non-nursing duties, including ward cleaning, patient transport and administrative ward duties, are no longer the responsibility of nurses. Within the nursing profession there are now specialists in a variety of areas such as intensive care, wound care, neurology and paediatric care. If we multiply this sort of specialisation of roles across the other health professionals – doctors, physiotherapists, occupational therapists, for example – then we can see that with so many different groups potentially involved in the care of a single patient there will inevitably be fragmentation in care arising from problems with effective communication and coordination of care [16].

The growth in specialisation also means that no one group ever has complete information about other workers' roles in patient care. As the management and care of patients is spread between so many health professional groups and departments, the information about a patient is often inaccurate or incomplete. The more complex and specialised the care requirements of a patient the more likely there will be errors in care, but even patients with minimal complexity are still at risk of an error of communication or coordination [11]. This potential risk is increased by the unique professional culture that operates in healthcare organisations, which is the focus of the next section.

Health professional culture

There are several features of the culture of healthcare professionals that are unique. The first is that the model of medical professional authority prevails within healthcare. We must emphasise here that what we are talking about is not the personal characteristics of any individual doctor, but rather the historical background in which medical practice has developed where doctors have considerable influence on the content of their own work (autonomy), over other health occupations (authority) and are accepted as institutionalised experts in all matters relating to health in wider society (sovereignty) [17–19].

This medical dominant culture impacts on the risk of errors occurring in several ways – firstly by nursing, other health professionals, and the general community accepting and reinforcing the idealistic professional philosophy of clinical perfection that has an expectation of error free performance [20, 21]. This type of culture inhibits error reporting and thus the opportunity to learn from mistakes. Secondly, the medical dominant culture gives rise to an authority gradient (one where people are reluctant to speak out for fear of negative consequences). This compromises effective teamwork and communication and is more likely to lead to errors as individuals are afraid to speak up when they can see a potential error and thus the opportunity to prevent the error is lost [20, 21].

A second feature of healthcare culture that makes it different to other organisations is that clinical staff providing care are working in a climate where the product (patients and families) they are dealing with is already flawed (patients are sick, families are grieving), or as an acceptable part of their role, they damage the product (surgical intervention, painful procedures) [22]. These professionals are accustomed to the outcome of their care not necessarily providing a perfect solution. They work daily in situations where people get sicker from chronic or terminal diseases, or where medication and treatments do not work. They work with patients and families to increase acceptance of suboptimal health status and support people as they learn to live (or die) with the results of traumatic injuries or acute and chronic diseases. Health professionals thus deal constantly with the results of life's inescapable and often painful events. To function effectively, health professionals must accept that in providing care, even when they are providing the best possible care, this may not result in a positive outcome for the patient. They therefore develop a tolerance for things going wrong or not being perfect [22].

Contrast this situation to other industries often compared to the health industry, for example the airline, oil or nuclear industries. These industries function in a safety paradigm of low tolerance for near misses, adverse events and poor outcomes [23]. Any flawed or damage product, once identified, acts as a trigger to review and thus reduce or prevent the likelihood of a repeat of the factors that led to the problem. If errors and incidents are to trigger the same immediate response within the healthcare arena, then the challenge is to find a way to increase health professionals' awareness to preventable adverse events and errors while not fracturing the coping mechanisms that allow them to accept inevitable poor clinical outcomes [22].

Complex systems and errors

Any patient entering a healthcare organisation will encounter many departments, systems, processes and different health professional specialists within a professional culture that is unique to healthcare. These will all contribute to a patient's episode of care. Many of these processes may not be obvious to the patient and, if something is not quite right in one of the processes, the end result may not affect the patient at all. However, if there are multiple things not quite right, the sum of these can lead to an error that directly affects the patient [21]. James Reason's Swiss Cheese model [8] is often used to describe this situation. The analogy of Swiss cheese is that the complexity and the number of processes, each of which has checks to prevent errors, provide protective layers (layers of Swiss cheese) for the patient. The assumption is that if one of these layers let an error through one of the holes, the next layer will stop the error. However, when the holes in the layers of cheese line up exactly, the errors are able to penetrate to the patient (see Figure 1.1). These holes in the layers are referred to as latent errors, as they are failures that occur removed in time and or space (blunt end) from the final end result (sharp end). As noted previously, the direct failure or end result of errors at multiple levels is called an active error [8, 9].

Defensive layers safeguarding patient

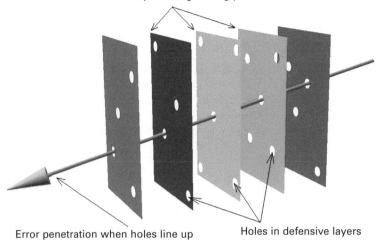

Error penetration when holes line up   Holes in defensive layers

Figure 1.1   Swiss Cheese model. Reproduced from *Human error: Models and management* by J. Reason in British Medical Journal v320 © 2000, with permission from BMJ Publishing Group Ltd

---

An example of a system gone wrong

To illustrate this take the example of a patient who was booked for surgery. When the patient was admitted to the ward there was another patient with the same surname on that ward. There is a ward policy that when two patients with surnames similar or the same are admitted to the ward, a red alert sticker 'patient with similar name' is placed on each patient's notes. However, the regular ward administration clerk was off sick and the replacement clerk did not know where the stickers were and so the alert sticker was not placed on the notes. When the theatre orderly arrived to transfer the patient to theatre, he went to the room allocated to the patient as identified on the theatre list and assisted the patient onto the trolley. The ward was very busy and so being helpful and hoping to save some time he retrieved the patient's notes from the office filing cabinet himself rather than waiting for the nurse to get these.

The ward practice was that the theatre orderly would assist the patient onto the trolley and then wait while a nurse retrieved that patient's notes and checked these with the patient ID bracelet. The ward nurse who was asked by the coordinator to accompany the patient to theatre saw that the theatre orderly had the notes in his hand and assumed that someone else had already checked these with the patient ID. The operating theatre was particularly busy and short staffed this day, consequently the student nurse was asked to check patients into the pre-anaesthetic room. When the patient arrived in the operating theatre, the student nurse confirmed the patient's name by asking them their surname. This matched the name on the notes. The student nurse was not aware that normal procedure required that the patient name is cross-checked by comparing the notes with the ID bracelet. Subsequently, it turned out that the wrong patient was operated on, as the patients with the same surname on the ward were mixed up.

If we relate this to the Swiss Cheese model – all of the processes and checks that are in place failed, thus the error of the wrong patient was able to penetrate to the patient with a disastrous result.

Exercise 1.2

Aim of the exercise: To identify the latent errors that may have contributed to the specific error that you identified in Exercise 1.1.

What to do:

1. Review the error and the contributing factors that you listed in the previous exercise. Think about the organisational systems and processes that may be involved 'behind the scenes' in the context of your error. Can you identify any aspects resulting from increased specialisation or health professional culture that may have contributed to the error? Add any further factors that you think may have contributed.
2. Now draw a rough sketch of the Swiss Cheese model. Label each slice of cheese with the latent error that penetrated the defences and resulted in the active error (what you actually did).
3. Discuss your example with friends or colleagues. Are there any similarities or differences with their examples?
4. Which items on the list grab your attention? What do these suggest to you that might be useful in your own work setting? Note these down also.
5. Compare your findings with the Exercise Feedback section at the end of the chapter.

This section has focused on some of the organisational factors that impact on the likelihood that an error will occur. Any combination of these factors can result in a cascade of latent factors that may result in an error provoking situation where the clinician at the coalface is more likely to make a mistake, slip, lapse or violation that results in an error. In the next section we will look briefly at how our understanding of how humans cognitively function can be utilised in the design of systems, processes, technology and machines to decrease the chance of mistakes happening. This is known as *human factors* [24, 25].

The Study of Human Factors

The study of human factors in healthcare is a relatively new area of research focusing on understanding how human fallibility is related to that ways people think and act and using that knowledge to design work systems, processes, technology, machines and the work environment that lessen the likelihood of errors [3]. Other industries such as the aviation, nuclear and space industries, as well as the military, have been using knowledge of human factors to design and improve systems and processes for many years [26]. Some of the solutions to error prone situations developed in these other industries are now being applied in healthcare. These system and process solutions can include such things as checklists, which reduce dependence on memory; simplifying and standardising procedures; double-checking procedures; and individual and team capacity building to raise awareness of human fallibility. These solutions, and others relating to system and process strategies, will be explored in the following chapters as they apply to specific error prone situations such as those involving consumers (Chapter 2), infection control (Chapter 3), medication administration (Chapter 4), teamwork and communication (Chapter 5) and individual vulnerability (Chapter 7).

Human factors principles can also be applied to the design of work environments, technology and machinery. This may include considering the design of visual and auditory displays and the usability of machinery, technology and computer software. Planning the design of workplaces, including lighting, noise levels, positioning of equipment and individual workspaces, to increase comfort and performance can significantly decrease the likelihood of error [3, 26]. This discipline of study is termed human factors engineering [20].

Some human factor engineering examples that focus on preventing slips, lapses and mistakes include:

- forcing functions that are designed to stop automatic options – for instance changing the threads on gas cylinders so that they cannot be connected to the wrong outlet on anaesthetic machines [20]
- designing medical machinery so data displays are easily visible from all angles and consistent with accepted standards (e.g. red for danger, green for ok) and alarms are of a tone easily heard and visualised
- setting the controls and display up in an uncluttered manner with a logical association between the two
- designing cable, tubing and other connections and fittings so that they will only fit into the correct outlet and the right way up
- ensuring knobs and switches cannot be inadvertently turned off or on by knocking them [10].

The opportunities for focusing on these types of solutions are endless, and it is more than likely that you have been interacting with human factors engineering design without realising. The next exercise is intended to identify some of the more common examples.

Exercise 1.3

Aim of the exercise: To identify examples of human factors engineering design.

What to do:

1. Read a selection of the articles and book sections below:

   - Gosbee, J., *Human factors engineering and patient safety,* Quality and Safety in Health Care 2002. 11: 352–354
   - Sawyer, D., *Do It By Design: An introduction to human factors in medical design,* 1996, US Department of Health & Human Services. Available at: www.fda.gov/downloads/ medicaldevices/deviceregulationandguidance/guidance documents/ucm095061.pdf.

2. Using the information from these and the previous section look at some of the common equipment that you work with or around your home and identify any human factors engineering designs that assist with the prevention of slips, lapses and mistakes.

3. Discuss your examples with colleagues.
4. Which aspects of the readings grabbed your attention? What do these suggest to you that might be useful in your own work setting? Note these down.
5. Compare your findings with the Exercise Feedback section at the end of the chapter.

Summary

This chapter has introduced you to patient safety concepts and the organisational and human factors that contribute to errors. We briefly introduced some organisational systems and processes that promote patient safety. The focus of the rest of the book is on specific strategies that should be used by healthcare organisations and health professionals to ensure that the care received by patients and their families is as safe as possible.

When an error happens in patient care it would be much simpler and easier to be able to identify the incompetent person who made the error and either send them for retraining or discipline them in some way. Both of these strategies may be required to make sure that the error never happens again! If it was a major error then it would be even easier to just fire them from the organisation, which absolutely removes the problem. However, while this sort of 'blaming and shaming' management of errors and adverse events may still be a reaction of some, the assumption that removing the person fixes the problem denies the organisation and others the opportunity to learn from the event. This learning from the event is far more likely to lessen the chances of the same error happening again. And, while an individual may be responsible for the error at face value, the organisation may have been complicit by virtue of the culture that it has fostered over the years leading up to the error. Removing the individual offender will not remove the potential for subsequent errors occurring with other staff.

The themes of this chapter relate to the WHO curriculum guideline topics of [27]:

• What is patient safety?
• Why human factors are important for patient safety
• Understanding systems and the complexity of care.

The Exercise Feedback below provides an overview of the key points of this chapter.

EXERCISE FEEDBACK

Exercise 1.1

There may be many contributing factors to why people make errors. These factors may be related to the way we think and process information, which in turn can be adversely influenced by physical, emotional or environmental pressures and the organisational systems and processes we are experiencing at the time of the error. These factors can include such things as:

- inadequate written or verbal communication
- lack of training
- distraction
- memory lapse
- poorly designed equipment
- poor teamwork
- lack of resources (e.g. equipment, policies, procedures, human resources)
- fatigue, sickness or stress
- noisy working environment
- other personal stresses (e.g. feeling unwell, family or financial pressures).

Exercise 1.2

Latent errors are decisions or processes that occur at the blunt end of care – that is, removed from where the actual error occurs at the point of care. The combination of latent errors is sometimes referred to as 'an accident waiting to happen'. In healthcare these can include such factors as:

- policy and/or managerial decisions on the levels of human and material resources
- policies and procedures not available to provide guidance
- inadequate education and training for role or task requirements
- poor design of equipment or work environment
- unsupportive team and work environment
- chaotic or complex work environment
- failure to undertake a risk assessment and plan accordingly.

Exercise 1.3

Human factors engineering design considers how human beings think and process information to make decisions about actions and incorporates this knowledge into the design of technology, machinery and environments to minimise the chance of errors. In this exercise you may have noted the following factors in the equipment you examined:

- on/off switch is obvious
- visual or audible cue that the equipment is on or off or about to be turned off
- alarms are easily heard and visualised and appropriately scaled from low level alarms to high level alarms
- alarm silence for critical functions cannot be turned off
- is the equipment intuitive to use?
- labels and displays are easily read from all angles
- obvious where and which way round leads, batteries and cables go
- link between control function and associated display function is obvious
- abbreviations, symbols and text should correspond to standard terminology
- switches and control knobs are placed in such a way as to allow easy user access but reduce the chance of unintentional initiation.

References

1. O'Leary, D. and L. Leape, *Teaching physicians to provide safe patient care*, in *Patient Safety Handbook*, B. Youngberg, ed. 2013, Maryland: James & Bartlett Learning.
2. Wilson, R., et al., *Patient safety in developing countries: Retrospective estimation of scale and nature of harm to patients in hospital*. BMJ, 2012. **344**: e832.
3. Carayon, P., ed. *Handbook of Human Factors and Ergonomics in Health Care and Patient Safety*. 2nd ed. *Human Factors and Ergonomics*, ed. G. Salvendy, 2012, Boca Raton, Florida: CRC Press.
4. de Vries, E., et al., *The incidence and nature of in-hospital adverse events: A systematic review*. Quality and Safety in Health Care, 2007. **17**(3): 216–223.
5. *WHO Draft Guidelines for Adverse Event Reporting Systems and Learning Systems*, 2005, Geneva: World Health Organization.
6. IOM, *To Err is Human: Building a safer health care system*, 2000, Washington, DC: National Academy Press.
7. Woods, D., et al., *Behind Human Error*, 2010, Farnham, Surrey: Ashgate Publishing.

8. Reason, J. *Human error: Models and management.* BMJ, 2000. **320**: 768–770.
9. Reason, J., *Beyond the organisational accident: The need for "error wisdom" on the frontline.* Quality and Safety in Health Care, 2004. **13**: 28–33.
10. Reynard, J., J. Reynolds, and P. Stevenson, *Practical Patient Safety,* 2009, Oxford: Oxford University Press.
11. Dekker, S., *A Field Guide to Understanding Human Error,* 2006, Aldershot, Hampshire: Ashgate Publishing.
12. Parker, D. and R. Lawton, *Psychological approaches to patient safety,* in *Patient Safety: Research into practice,* K. Walshe and R. Boaden, eds. 2006, Maidenhead, Berkshire: Open University Press: 31–40.
13. Powell, A., R. Rushmer, and H. Davies, *Effective quality improvement: BPR.* British Journal of Healthcare Management, 2009. **15**(4): 166–171.
14. Rasmussen, J. and A. Jensen, *Mental procedures in real life tasks: A case study of electronic trouble shooting.* Ergonomics, 1974. **17**(17): 293–307.
15. Reason, J., *The Human Contribution: Unsafe acts, accidents and heroic recoveries,* 2008, Farnham, Surrey: Ashgate Publishing.
16. Runciman, W., A. Merry, and M. Walton, *Safety and Ethics in Healthcare: A guide to getting it right,* 2007, Aldershot, Hampshire: Ashgate Publishing.
17. Willis, E., *Introduction: Taking stock of medical dominance.* Health Sociology Review, 2006. **15**: 421–431.
18. Long, D., et al., *The (im)possibilities of clinical democracy.* Health Sociology Review, 2006. **15**: 506–519.
19. Carroll, J. and M. Quijada, *Redirecting traditional professional values to support safety: Changing organisational culture in health care.* Quality and Safety in Health Care, 2004. **13**: 16–21.
20. Wachter, R., *Understanding Patient Safety.* 2nd ed. 2012, San Francisco: McGraw-Hill.
21. IOM, *Keeping Patients Safe: Transforming the work environment of nurses,* 2004, Washington, DC: National Academy Press.
22. Walshe, K. and S. Shortell, *When things go wrong: How health care organisations deal with major failures.* Health Affairs, 2004. **23**: 103–111.
23. Schulman, P., *General attributes of safe organisations.* Quality and Safety in Health Care, 2004. **13**: 39–44.
24. Powell, A., R. Rushmer, and H. Davies, *Effective quality improvement: Recognising the challenges.* British Journal of Healthcare Management, 2009. **15**(1): 17–21.
25. Powell, A., R. Rushmer, and H. Davies, *Effective quality improvement: Conclusion.* British Journal of Healthcare Management, 2009. **15**(8): 374–379.
26. Proctor, R. and T. Van Zandt, *Human Factors in Simple and Complex Systems,* 2008, Boca Raton, Florida: CRC Press.
27. *WHO Patient Safety Curriculum Guide: Multi-professional edition,* 2011, Geneva: World Health Organization.

2

Engaging Patients in the Safety Agenda

Introduction

It is quite remarkable that, when talking about patient safety, the majority of improvement strategies target health professionals and healthcare organisations. It appears as if the patient is merely an inactive participant in this complex world of healthcare. Much of the literature focuses on patient safety from the health professionals' perspective. The patients' perspective and the role that patients may have in patient safety initiatives are not given very much attention.

This is not new: in a stinging attack on the medicalised healthcare system Illich [1] wrote about the notion of iatrogenesis – the physician induced damage caused to people seeking care, help and treatment, which in his view reached epidemic proportions several decades ago. A major determinant of iatrogenic care lay in the inappropriate levels of power and control in the hands of the medical profession. He cautioned that:

A professional and physician-based health care system which has grown beyond tolerable bounds is sickening for these reasons: it must produce clinical damages which outweigh its potential benefits; it cannot but enhance even as it obscures the political conditions which rendered society unhealthy; and it tends to expropriate the power of the individual to heal himself and to shape his or her environment. [1: 9]

While the account offered by Illich had a distinctly medical emphasis the reality is that all health professionals run the risk of doing harm while intending to do good. Allied health workers, nurses, psychologists, pharmacists, dentists, and alternative therapists can inadvertently injure a patient through poor treatment or advice. As health professionals it is hard to contemplate this but the evidence is clear and unequivocal.

If professional power is at work here then it is one of several issues that need consideration. The term 'health professional' implies expertise and knowledge that is not widely held and is to some extent investing health professionals with a level of power and control over those who seek out our help. Paradoxically, a significant amount of time and effort these days is (or should be) focused on helping people and patients to become responsible for their own health and decisions about their lives and treatment options. This approach is about enabling people to be empowered, although not everyone will embrace this sort of thinking. There is a tension in the health professional role here that needs to be acknowledged. Being a professional means having expertise and skills that people sometimes need but it also means being influential in helping people to make their own decisions rather than directing or instructing them from a traditional position of power enshrined in a specific role within the healthcare system.

The notion of iatrogenic care is an important one as it highlights the issue of patient safety framed within the more traditional and evolving roles and expectations of health professionals and healthcare consumers. Increasing numbers of patients and their families want to be actively involved in managing their health [2]. As well, health professionals are starting to understand that with the increasing complexity and fragmentation of care processes, patients need to be more involved in patient safety.

This chapter explores patient safety with an emphasis on the patients' viewpoint – especially their role in the prevention and management of errors. The placing of this chapter as the second one in the book is in deliberate recognition of the fact that patients are often the last people to be considered in the patient safety concept, yet their contribution (apart from being victims) is invaluable in the prevention of errors. We will begin this chapter with a story.

Kathleen's story

Familiarity can breed lazy thinking ... .

Kathleen is 85 years old. All of her life from a very young age she worked hard. She subscribed to the belief that 'the harder you work the luckier you get' and expected others to do likewise in all walks of life. She smoked cigarettes from a young age too and over the last decade or so suffered from chronic infections and breathing difficulties. As she aged she lost weight and became a pale reflection of her old energetic self. Her brain and awareness of the world continued to be razor sharp. Her ill health meant that she had frequent meetings with her GP who seemed like a genuine caring person. Often he told Kathleen what a 'marvellous' woman she was for her age. She was always appreciative and uncritical of the care she received and never complained. She was of the post-war generation with a highly independent spirit.

For over a year now Kathleen had complained of pains in her abdomen intermittently and the sensation of a 'lump' but the GP told her it was probably a 'fatty deposit'. No investigations were done. Recently she began feeling sick and needed an antiemetic. After two weeks these symptoms were getting progressively worse and the antiemetic provided only temporary relief. Most recently she was so ill she 'felt she was going to die' and her daughter called out the locum GP. After listening to her story he rushed her to hospital and as luck would have it she was seen by a surgical team almost immediately. In spite of her medical history, surgery was done to repair a strangulated hernia. The team leader told her that she almost died. Kathleen made a good recovery but is very angry now that nobody from the healthcare team bothered to investigate her symptoms because she was 'too old and familiar'. If they had done, all of the pain and suffering could have been avoided.

Of course, in the story above the obvious problem is delayed diagnosis leading to an emergency situation for Kathleen. However, before we criticise the GP involved we need to remember the discussion from the previous chapter about how humans make mistakes. You will have noted that when we are consciously processing information to come up with solutions to problems our default is to come up with an answer that has worked before using stored information. Either confirmation bias or frequency gambling bias could well have been part of the decision made by the GP that Kathleen's abdominal pain was not sinister. There may have been other factors that influenced this particular scenario. There may have been opportunities missed to involve Kathleen more in her care, or factors that acted as barriers to the GP really 'hearing' what Kathleen was saying to him about her abdominal pain. These factors make up the slices of 'Swiss cheese' (see Chapter 1) that allowed the error of delayed diagnosis to penetrate to the patient. In this chapter we will explore these factors – the role patients and their families can play in preventing errors – and then we will focus on the barriers that make it difficult for patients to be involved in their care.

Finally we will look at strategies to involve patients. Don't forget Kathleen, as we will return to her story later in the chapter.

Opportunities for Patient Involvement in Care

Have you ever played that game of Chinese whispers where a message is whispered from person to person and then the original message is compared to the final message? It can be very interesting. In the majority of cases the message at the end is quite different, and in some instances the final message bears no resemblance at all to the original. This is especially so if the message was technical and complicated. Relate this to the situation we talked about in the previous chapter where there are so many health professionals caring for any single patient through their episode of care. The chances of an error in information transfer between different health professionals are high. This is further complicated when the care spans several sectors such as primary care, acute care and chronic care.

Patients and their families have a huge investment in wanting the best possible care and in us (healthcare workers) getting it right. It is important to realise that patients are the only people who are there for the whole episode of their care, from beginning to end. They are therefore in the unique position of being able to tell you what happened and when, in terms of care given or omitted. It makes sense, then, to harness this investment and knowledge to ensure that patients receive the best possible care by partnering with them and their families to plan and deliver that care. Patients can contribute in many areas throughout their care episode. This includes helping towards an accurate diagnosis: patients and their families can provide clinicians with information about their illness (symptoms, duration, onset, location, alleviating or precipitating factors, etc.) that will increase the likelihood of a correct diagnosis [3].

Patients and families should be involved in decisions about their treatment options. They are the real experts in their lives. They are absolutely familiar with their own circumstances, values and preferences. Once they have been given accurate information about the harms and benefits of treatment options, the decision about treatment choices should be shared between patients and the clinicians. Studies have consistently demonstrated that this type of shared decision making is far more likely to lead to compliance with treatment regimes, especially with chronic illness, and also that patients are less likely to accept ineffective or risky procedures [4–7]. However, there will be some people who will still want to defer to the health experts – those who are older or who find making decisions about treatment options very difficult. This perspective too needs to be accommodated.

Patients who are informed about their medication regime, including expected action and possible side effects, are then able to inform staff about their response to the medication. If patients understand the processes of administration such as dosage, frequency and the checks made when clinicians administer medication, then they are able to alert staff if they feel there are changes from the expected routine. Considering that medication errors are involved in a significant number of adverse events, the potential role that patients and their families can play in preventing these cannot be overstated [3]. We delve more into medication incidents in Chapter 4.

While the practice of patients having access to their medical records is uncommon, the benefits of it becoming more widespread would be two-fold: it would allow patients to check the accuracy of the records as well as give them a greater understanding of their health status. Studies have provided evidence of these – one study demonstrated that when patients viewed their medical records 30 per cent of those records were incorrect [8].

Although patients suffer considerable psychological trauma following an adverse event, they want to know what happened and what can be done to prevent it happening again [6, 9]. Open disclosure is a process whereby patients and their families are told when an adverse event has taken place, and is included in the process of trying to understand the factors that led to the adverse event. The open disclosure principles have been adopted as part of the patient safety framework by WHO [10], and many countries including Australia, the United Kingdom, Canada and New Zealand have adopted policies supporting this process. Importantly, this open disclosure process provides not only closure for the patients but also the opportunity for health professionals and organisations to learn from patients and families, whose viewpoint can be used to inform the development of strategies to prevent similar incidents happening again [11, 12].

There are many opportunities for patients and their families to be involved in their care. However, it must be remembered that although it makes very good sense for patients to be actively involved, the responsibility for ensuring patient safety belongs to the clinicians and the healthcare organisations in which the care is delivered. In some circumstances it is important for patients to follow instructions to ensure safety (e.g. medication adherence or pre-operative preparation). It is important to remember then that patients are the experts in their own lives – it is vital for the health worker to remember this and to learn the skills required for working in partnership with the patient (and family) to ensure that all relevant information is elicited and explored during two way interactions. Such a process will engage patients fully and minimise risk.

In the next section we will discuss the barriers to patients and their families being actively involved in their care. But firstly we suggest you complete the following exercise.

Exercise 2.1

Aim of the exercise: To identify the barriers to involving patients in care.

What to do:

1. Talk to at least three people asking them to describe an experience as a patient or as a family member supporting a patient. It doesn't have to be an experience where the person was hospitalised – it could be an experience with their GP, community health nurse or a visit to an outpatient clinic. Complete the table below for each person you talk to. Try to keep the conversation reasonably 'light' – maybe use examples like a sporting injury, heavy cold, chest infection, etc.

Patient or family members felt they were ...	Yes or No
Involved in reaching an accurate diagnosis	
Given enough information to give informed consent about treatments and procedures	
Informed about the timing of doses, actions and side effects of any medication regime	
Asked to check the accuracy of their medical record	
Asked if they identified any errors in their treatment	
Asked if there were things they did not understand	
Treated with respect	
Listened to	
Given an opportunity to ask questions	

2. Now for all of the 'No' answers make a list of the possible reasons the patient (or family member) was not involved.

3. Talk about your answers with other people and see if you can add any other reasons to your list.
4. Review your list after you have read the next section and see if you can add anything to it. Consider these questions: What particular items on the list stand out? How might these be added to your own efforts to engage patients and families more constructively? Will you need to change your behaviour in any way?
5. Compare your findings with the Exercise Feedback section at the end of the chapter.

Barriers to Patient Involvement in Care

In the previous section we established that engaging patients in their care is an excellent strategy to reduce errors and adverse outcomes – especially if patients understand fully what is required of them and wish to be active participants in their care and treatment. So, if it makes sense to involve people in their care why doesn't this happen more often? In this section we will talk about the common barriers to patient involvement.

A significant barrier to patient involvement is that many patients and their families are not in a position to understand fully their care or their care choices. There are several reasons for this – one is that their illness can lead to very strong feelings of anxiety and uncertainty which can prevent a person from engaging in the process in a confident and constructive manner. Many people assume the sick role, one of passivity, where they willingly hand over responsibility for decisions about their care to the experts [13]. You may have come across people in your care who openly declare, 'I don't really want to know all the details ... how long will I be off work and when can I start training again'? Such an approach is fine up to a point, but can be the root cause of errors and poor outcomes.

A lack of understanding can also occur because of language and cultural barriers. If patients do not have this understanding then the likelihood of them becoming active participants in their care is very low [3].

To overcome language barriers many health services have a translator service available, either in person or using telephone access.

However, these services are under-utilised, in both hospital and community settings. The need for the translator service may not be obvious to the health professional until after the encounter with the patient has begun – and then the service takes time to organise and access. The use of translators is not without some challenges however, especially where cultural issues are concerned, and it is important to try to use trained translators rather than family or staff members who may be more readily available.

Benson and Thistlethwaite [14] introduced the Cultural Awareness Tool for health practitioners working across cultures. It is underpinned by research and draws on their personal and professional experiences. The Cultural Awareness Tool comprises a number of questions designed to elicit and explore client problems in a culturally sensitive way, using stories as the primary vehicle of communication. The tool includes questions like:

• What do you think caused your problem?
• How severe is your illness?
• What do you fear most about it?
• How is your community helping you?

Many different cultural factors can curtail a person's ability to engage with professional services. Poor language skills, social isolation, prohibitive costs, restrictions about women's movements in public, and cultural obligations that women see a female professional will all influence people's choices and decisions about health related actions.

Another barrier to patients being involved in their care is low health literacy. Health literacy is defined by Wachter [12] as 'the degree to which individuals have the capacity to obtain, process and understand basic health information and services to make appropriate health decisions' [12: 373].

Written material such as pamphlets and other reading matter provide an opportunity to assist patients and families to increase their knowledge and understanding. It is vital, however, that this reading matter is suitable in terms of target language, terminology and cultural appropriateness [15].

Patients should also be encouraged to search out their own information via libraries, special interest groups and, if available, the internet – the reality is that often patients and families get more information from these resources than from their health professionals [16]. Recognising this – and the fact that information from these sources may not always be of high quality – it is important that patients and families have the opportunity to ask questions about the content and the treatment options described. A well-informed patient can alter the power dynamic that shapes a professional relationship and may lead to some health professionals feeling uncomfortable and challenged [4, 17, 18]. However, as health professionals we need to appreciate that many people will come to us better informed through the internet than ever before. We need to embrace these new technologies and ensure those internet sites sourced by patients are of the highest quality – ideally those we use ourselves in our work.

Patients need to feel comfortable talking with health professionals. They need the time and skills to be able to read information, access healthcare when they need it, and understand their treatment plan. Health professionals can help with health literacy by encouraging patients to ask questions and digest information, making sure they are given adequate unhurried time to do so [15, 19].

Cultural barriers that exist within healthcare – both professional and organisational – act as an enormous block for patients striving to question or challenge those who are caring for them. In the main, health professionals espouse a patient centred care philosophy, but they do not always practise the philosophy. The assertive, challenging patient, for example, may be viewed negatively, and perceived as lacking an understanding of the complexity of healthcare delivery. This professional culture marginalises patients and families and discourages active involvement [6, 16, 20–23].

There is increasing recognition of this barrier to patient involvement, and there have been many campaigns to encourage patients to raise any concerns or ask questions about the care they are getting [4]. However, it is probably no surprise that several studies have found that even well-informed patients and families may be unwilling to question healthcare staff about the care they are receiving [24, 25]. Overall it is clear that even where patients are given practical evidence about patient safety issues, and things they can do to help prevent errors, they do not feel 'empowered' to question health professionals' actions. To address this, all health professional staff need to receive training and education to give them insight into how their behaviours and those of other health professionals can impact negatively on patients' active involvement in their own care and treatment [19].

The reticence on the part of patients and families to ask questions or their inability to process the information being given to them can also be a result of the perceived busyness of those caring for them. With the average GP consultation being about 8 minutes, and the increasing activity and acuity across all domains of health, many patients do not feel it is appropriate to interrupt or take more time to ask questions or discuss in detail those things that are concerning them [5, 26–28].

Patients will remain passive recipients of care if they feel, or if they fear, that their care will be compromised if they ask questions, challenge health professionals or raise issues of concern in regards to unsafe care. Fear of retribution of, at the very least, poor care is very real [5]. Health professionals have to understand what it is like for patients to be in an unfamiliar place, worried and unsure about what is wrong with them and what the treatment might mean to them with their particular set of personal circumstances [12].

Exercise 2.2

Aim of the exercise: To identify the opportunities and barriers to involving Kathleen more in her care that may have prevented the delayed diagnosis. You may wish to review James Reason's Swiss Cheese model described in Chapter 1 before you start.

What to do:

1. Reread Kathleen's story at the beginning of this chapter. Now make a list of the opportunities missed to involve Kathleen in her care and the barriers that may have prevented this involvement.
2. Draw a rough sketch of the Swiss Cheese model. Label each slice of cheese with the errors you have identified that penetrated the defences and resulted in the misdiagnosis.
3. Discuss your example with friends or colleagues. Are there any similarities or differences with their examples?
4. Which items on the list grab your attention? What do these suggest to you that might be useful in your own work setting? Note these down also.
5. Compare your findings with the Exercise Feedback section at the end of the chapter.

Strategies to Involve Patients in Their Own Care

It is highly likely that if patients had less trust in the healthcare system and in healthcare workers they would be far more willing to be active participants in their care. The key message for patients and families is that:

- medicine and healthcare is not an exact science
- the health professionals caring for them are human and will make mistakes
- healthcare choices are not necessarily yes/no choices but rather weighing up the best choice to suit the patient and their circumstances.

Until the general public understands the message about the fallibility of healthcare professionals and the healthcare system there will be no significant push from the community to change the status quo. An appreciation of this fallibility is important in encouraging active rather than passive roles [5].

Patients and their families can only be involved in the planning of their care if they have knowledge and understanding of their treatment options, care and ongoing monitoring requirements, and awareness that they have choices. So how can this be achieved?

It is important firstly to understand the patients' perspective on what may increase active participation. When patients and their families are asked what is important to them in this regard the following factors stand out: patient knowledge; explicit encouragement of patient participation by physicians; appreciation of the patient's responsibility and right to play an active role in decision making; awareness of choice; and time (not feeling rushed when talking to the health professional) [3–5, 16, 18, 24, 29]. You will note that three of these factors (explicit encouragement of patient participation by physicians, appreciation of the patient's responsibility and right to play an active role in decision making, and time) require specific behaviours from health professionals rather than patients. We believe awareness of these is vital if patients are truly going to be partners in care and their potential to improve safety is to be realised.

So, patients must be included in discussions about their condition and treatment. The medical, nursing and other healthcare staff should use terminology that can be understood by the patient. These interactions need to be in an environment that is comfortable, where the patient feels safe psychologically, emotionally and socially to ask questions, and at a time when the patient is able to 'hear' what is being said, rather than when they are in crisis [3, 5, 27].

Exercise 2.3

Aim of the exercise: To understand patients' experiences.

What to do:

1. Read the following letter sourced from the *WHO Patient Safety Curriculum Guide: Multi-professional edition* [10]. The letter provides a patient's perspective on her hospital experience.

   I'm Alice, 25 years old. I had abdominal pain for six days and I was really frightened because my sister started a year ago with similar symptoms and now has intestinal cancer and is under a very aggressive treatment.

   I decided to go alone to the hospital in order not to scare the whole family. I arrived at the hospital early in the morning. I didn't know exactly what to do or who to see; it was my first time at the hospital. Everybody looked in a hurry and they did not look very friendly. Some of them looked as frightened as I was.

   I took a deep breath and asked a young lady who looked at me and smiled as if she knew where the gastrointestinal department was located. She laughed a little and said, 'I'm a medical student and I'm lost too. Let's try together to find it, I have to go to the same place too'. She said, 'Why don't we go to the information office?' I thought it was a good idea, and all of a sudden I started to feel in some way protected. A person I considered to be a health-care professional was with me.

   We arrived at the information office to find it was crowded with a lot of people shouting, some of them angry. There was only one person providing information. Lucy, the medical student said, 'I do not think we will get anywhere if we try to get information here'. I thought we could follow the signals I had seen at the main entrance. I said, 'Let's go'.

   After walking through the crowd, we arrived at the main entrance. We finally arrived at the gastrointestinal department. Lucy said, 'Oh, yes, this is the place, ask the nurse over there; I should go to take my class, good luck'.

   The nurse told me that I shouldn't come directly to the gastrointestinal department, that I should go to the emergency department and they would decide about my condition. So, I had to return to the emergency room. When I arrived, plenty of people were waiting; they told me I would have to wait. 'You should have come earlier', the nurse said (I arrived early!!).

   A general practitioner eventually saw me and ordered X-rays and lab examinations. Nobody said anything and no explanations were provided to me. At that moment I was more scared than when I woke up with the pain.

   I was at the hospital all day going from one place to another. At the end of the day, a doctor came and told me in few words you are OK, there is nothing to worry about, and I started 'breathing' again.

I would like to say to the hospital authorities that they should realize that every person coming to the hospital, even if they do not have any important disease, is feeling stressed and often unwell. We need friendly people taking care of us, ones who try to understand our story and why we feel so bad. We need clear communication between health-care workers and patients. We need clear information on how we should use the hospital facilities in order to make best use of them. I understand that you cannot cure everybody – unfortunately you are not Gods – but I am sure that you could be friendlier to patients. Doctors and nurses have the incredible power that only with his/her words, gestures and comprehension of the patient situation, they can make a patient feel secure and relieved.

Please do not forget this power so incredibly useful for those human beings who enter your hospital.

With all my respect,
Alice

Reproduced with kind permission of WHO.

2. Make a list of the positives and the negatives of Alice's experience.
3. Now imagine that we are getting the chance to rerun the whole scenario again and you are in the shoes of each of the health professionals that Alice comes in contact with. Write down what attitudes and behaviours you would change to improve Alice's experience and truly treat her as a partner in her own care.
4. Identify some potential errors that would be avoided with the changed behaviours you have described.
5. Discuss your findings with other colleagues. Are there other things that they identify that need improvement?
6. Compare your findings with the Exercise Feedback section at the end of the chapter.

What Can You as an Individual Health Practitioner Do?

As we have become more aware that we must partner with patients if we are to make the healthcare we deliver safer and improve outcomes, many initiatives have been developed, at both national policy and organisational levels. You will learn about several of these in the coming chapters. However, the individual health practitioner must also look to their own behaviour and identify those things they can do to ensure they actively engage with patients and families to involve them in choices and decisions about care.

The following list of behaviours has been gleaned from several different sources [10–12, 17, 18], and identifies the competencies needed by individual practitioners if they are to meaningfully partner with patients:

- actively encourage patients and families to share information
- show empathy, honesty and respect for patients and families
- communicate effectively (listen as well as talk!)
- ensure patients understand and are involved in the decision about treatments
- show respect for religious, cultural and individual preferences
- guide patients to suitable sources of health information
- help patients understand how to manage their own health condition
- check that the patient has understood – don't assume that they have.

Overall the most important thing is to tell patients what is happening. Use every interaction with a patient as an opportunity to inform them about what is going on, and explain each step of their treatment. For the health professional this may seem like endless repetition; for the patient it is precious information to help them build understanding of their care.

Your interactions with a patient will be more meaningful if you discuss with them their preferences for receiving information, rather than making assumptions about the medium they may prefer. There are many options available in today's technical world, including on-line information, written information, videos or digital recordings as well as the more traditional pamphlets, support groups and face-to-face discussions.

Actively encourage patients to voice their ideas, and expectations about their options for treatment. Discuss their choices in an open and respectful manner supported by the evidence. Consider that the patient's lifestyle, values and social situation may be impacting on their decisions about treatment, and respect the choices they make without overlaying your own preferences on what you think might be the best course of action [30].

As well, patients can be encouraged to highlight areas where they perceive there may be errors – or the potential for errors – in their care, for example incorrect or late medications, wrong procedures, clinicians not washing hands before undertaking care. However, studies have shown that patients are reluctant to raise issues of poor care or possible error [4], so as a clinician you must be quite explicit in telling the patient that it is okay to voice concerns and that doing so will not affect their ongoing care.

Patients can be encouraged to take part in their care, ask questions and raise concerns, but significant participation will not occur unless health professionals value patient involvement and contribution in more than a symbolic way, and appreciate the important impact of involvement in determining better outcomes for the patient. This also involves recognising that patients' experiences provide a unique window for health professionals to help them understand what it is like to be a patient undergoing treatment and making choices – but these experiences must be viewed as valuable if they are going to inform a positive culture that truly recognises that patients are partners in their own care. Indeed, this level of partnership appears to be a prerequisite for achieving informed consent.

Summary

This chapter has focused on the potential to engage patients as active and well-informed participants in their care and to use this as a strategy to prevent errors and decrease adverse events. At the start of the chapter a quote from Illich's 1976 book demonstrated that patients suffering adverse events as a result of their treatment is not a new concept. However, the current thinking now emphasises that it is an important role of health professionals to understand the patient viewpoint and to recognise the advantages this gives us in terms of achieving the goal of patient safety.

The themes of this chapter relate to the WHO curriculum guideline topic of [31]:

- Engaging with patients and carers.

The Exercise Feedback below provides an overview of the key points of this chapter.

EXERCISE FEEDBACK

Exercise 2.1

The barriers that can hinder active involvement of patients in their care include the following:

- patients may take on the passive 'sick role'
- language and cultural barriers
- uncomfortable relationship with health professionals involved in their care
- health professionals' culture of being the experts
- patients uncomfortable about challenging and asking questions of the health professional
- time constraints in the interactions with health professionals.

Exercise 2.2

In this story about misdiagnosis, human fallibility and the way people process information may well have been a major factor at the sharp end of care. However, the latent factors may have been:

- limited time for consultations
- lack of training and education for the GP to provide understanding about cognitive biases such as confirmation bias and frequency gambling bias
- not involving the patient's family in discussions which may have helped with an early diagnosis
- not seeking feedback from previous adverse events similar to this that may have provided a learning opportunity.

Exercise 2.3

The behaviours required of health professionals if patients are to feel empowered to be partners in their healthcare include:

- actively encourage patients and families to share information
- show empathy, honesty and respect for patients and families
- communicate effectively (listen as well as talk!)
- ensure patients understand and are involved in the decision about treatments
- show respect for religious, cultural and individual preferences

- guide patients to suitable sources of health information
- help patients understand how to manage their own health condition
- check that the patient has understood – don't assume that they have.

Health professionals can provide a climate that is more likely to encourage patient participation by doing the following:

- Ensuring that they constantly tell patients what is happening, how it is happening and why it is happening that way. What is ordinary to the health professional is often totally new to the patient who may have no idea what is happening and need help to understand the experience.
- Encouraging patients to report errors and raise concerns about their care. When they do, ensure that the first reaction is not a defensive one but rather one where the patient is recognised as a partner in care for raising the issue.
- Genuinely seeking understanding of the patient perspective as a foreigner navigating a system in a strange land where they do not speak the language or understand the culture.

References

1. Illich, I. *Medical Nemesis: The expropriation of health*, 1976, New York: Pentheon Books.
2. Lawton, R., et al., *Development of an evidence-based framework of factors contributing to patient safety incidents in hospital settings: A systematic review.* BMJ Quality & Safety, 2012. **21**: 369–380.
3. Ellins, J. and A. Coulter, *The patient's role in preventing errors and promoting safety*, in *Health Care Errors and Patient Safety*, B. Hurwitz and A. Sheikh, eds. 2009, Oxford: Blackwell Publishing.
4. Davis, R., M. Koutantji, and C. Vincent, *How willing are patients to question healthcare staff on issues related to the quality and safety of their healthcare: An exploratory study.* Quality and Safety in Health Care, 2008. **17**: 90–96.
5. Fraenkel, L. and S. McGraw, *What are the essential elements to enable patient participation in medical decision making?* Society of General Internal Medicine, 2006. **22**: 614–619.
6. Vincent, C. and A. Coulter, *Patient safety: What about the patient?* Quality and Safety in Health Care, 2002. **11**: 76–80.
7. Wolff, A. and S. Taylor, *Enhancing Patient Safety: A practical guide to improving quality and safety in hospitals*, 2009, Sydney: MJA Books.
8. Coulter, A., *After Bristol: Putting patients at the centre.* Quality and Safety in Health Care, 2002. **11**: 186–188.
9. Vincent, C., ed. *Clinical Risk Management: Enhancing patient safety.* 2nd ed. 2001, London: BMJ Books.

10. *WHO Patient Safety Curriculum Guide: Multi-professional edition,* 2011, Geneva: World Health Organization.
11. Iedema, R., R. Sorenson, and D. Piper, *Open disclosure: A review of the literature,* 2008, Australian Commission on Quality and Safety in Healthcare.
12. Wachter, R., *Understanding Patient Safety.* 2nd ed. 2012, San Francisco: McGraw-Hill.
13. Frosch, D., et al., *Authoritarian physicians and patients' fear of being labeled "difficult" among key obstacles to shared decision making.* Health Affairs, 2012. **31**(5): 1030–1038.
14. Benson, J. and J. Thistlethwaite, *Mental Health Across Cultures: A practical guide for health professionals,* 2009, Oxford: Radcliffe Publishing.
15. Prabhakar, H., et al., *Introducing standardized "readbacks" to improve patient safety in surgery: A prospective survey in 92 providers at a public safety-net hospital.* BMC Surgery, 2012. **12**: 8.
16. Hallisy, J., *The Empowered Patient,* 2008, San Francisco: Bold Spirit Press.
17. Mahajan, R., *Critical incident reporting and learning.* British Journal of Anaesthetics, 2010. **105**(1): 69–75.
18. Conway, J., et al., *Partnering with Patients and Families to Design a Patient- and Family-Centered Health Care System: A roadmap for the future,* 2006, Bethesda, USA: Institute for Family-Centred Care & Institute for Health Care Improvement.
19. Wright, S. and M. Fallacaro, *Predictors of situation awareness in student registered nurse anaesthetists.* AANA Journal, 2011. **79**(6): 484–490.
20. Dekker, S., *Patient Safety: A human factors approach,* 2011, Boca Raton, Florida: CRC Press.
21. Douglas, N., J. Robinson, and K. Fahy, *Inquiry into Obstetrics and Gynaecological Services at King Edward Memorial Hospital 1990–2000: Final report,* 2001, Perth, Western Australia: Government of Western Australia.
22. Johnson, A. and B. Beacham, *Concerns about being a Health Consumer Representative.* Australian Journal of Primary Care, 2006. **12**(3): 94.
23. Mahler, J., *Organisational Learning at NASA: The Challenger and Columbia accidents,* 2009, Washington, DC: Georgetown University Press.
24. Bismark, M., et al., *Relationship between complaints and quality of care: A descriptive analysis of non-complainants following adverse events.* Quality and Safety in Health Care, 2005. **15**(1): 17–22.
25. Gallagher, T. and M. Lucas, *Should we disclose harmful medical errors to patients? If so, how?* Journal of Clinical Outcomes Management, 2005. **12**(5): 253–259.
26. Dunn, N., *Commentary: Patient centred care: Timely but is it practical?* BMJ, 2002. **324**(7338): 651.
27. Frampton, S. and P. Charmel, *Putting Patients First: Best practices in patient-centred care.* 2nd ed. 2009, San Francisco: Jossey-Bass.
28. Towle, A. and W. Godolphin, *Framework for teaching and learning informed shared decision making.* BMJ, 1999. **319**(7212): 761–766.
29. Khadra, M., *The Patient,* 2009, Sydney: Random House.
30. Schuster, P. and L. Nykolyn, *Communication for Nurses,* 2010, Philadelphia: F.A. Davis.
31. *WHO Patient Safety Curriculum Guide: Multi-professional edition,* 2011, Geneva: World Health Organization.

3

Healthcare Acquired Infections

Introduction

The occurrence of healthcare acquired infections (HAIs) is high across all healthcare settings in both developing and developed countries – so much so that health professionals can become desensitised to the frequency of these events. The resulting mortality and morbidity for patients is enormous; length of stay increases dramatically and the cost of the episode of care can increase exponentially, both in financial terms and in terms of the human costs [1]. There has been a huge amount of research into identifying risk profiles of patients and the clinical settings in which HAIs are more likely to occur. Moreover, many evidence based care protocols have been developed to lessen the likelihood of HAIs. However, there is mounting evidence that the risk assessment tools and prevention strategies for these types of incidents are not being universally applied [2].

Prevention of HAIs requires continual vigilance and the use of routine tasks performed diligently and repeatedly. However, these routines do not enjoy the glamour and interest of many other clinical interventions and thus they can become of low priority. Making an impact on the incidence of these particular adverse events requires a commitment from all health professionals.

This chapter will review the evidence behind the prevention strategies that health practitioners should be implementing, and championing, within their own care contexts. We will begin the chapter with some background information about HAIs.

Background

A healthcare acquired infection (HAI) is defined as infection that occurs in a patient while they are being cared for that was not present

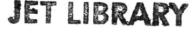

or incubating when the person was admitted to the healthcare facility [1]. Hospital associated infections, hospital acquired infection and nosocomial infections are other terms that are in common usage to describe HAIs, but these terms do not necessarily encompass the range of clinical settings covered by the term HAIs.

Since the 1950s there has been a significant amount of research into the prevention of HAIs. Many of the evidence based prevention strategies are simple to institute, but despite this HAIs remain one of the commonest adverse events experienced by patients [1]. A WHO report showed that across all four WHO regions (Europe, Eastern Mediterranean, South East Asia and the Western Pacific) the average rate of HAIs was 8.7 per cent [1]. In Australia and the United States the rates are estimated to be between 5 and 10 per cent [3]. In the UK there is not a national surveillance programme to monitor the incidence of all HAIs, but the rate is likely to be similar to other developed countries [4, 5]. HAIs have a substantial impact not only on patients and their families but also on the length of stay (LOS) and the cost of patient care. Studies estimate that the LOS can increase by on average 8–9 days with costs of care increased by 24 per cent [1, 5].

Although we are principally looking at developed countries in this book it is important to understand that HAIs are a significant problem also in developing countries. In fact developing countries carry a disproportionate burden in terms of HAIs, with some studies showing a prevalence rate of 15.5 per cent in hospitals, 47.9 per cent in ICUs and 5.6 per cent in surgical procedures [6]. Although there are limited studies, it is suggested these high rates are related to factors such as environmental hygiene, poor infrastructure, understaffing, overcrowding, lack of knowledge about infection control principles in healthcare workers, prolonged use of invasive devices, and reuse of supplies such as needles and gloves [6]. Hand hygiene is considered to be the single most important strategy to reduce HAIs, yet in developing countries the observance of this is noted to be lacking, with some studies showing rates as low as 20 per cent [6, 7].

HAIs are transmitted in two ways, namely endogenous or exogenous spread. Endogenous spread occurs when the microorganisms which are normally present in different body sites such as the nose, mouth or gastrointestinal tract are transferred from one part of the patient's body to another which normally is not colonised by them, and so results in an infection. This is most often via healthcare workers' hands. Exogenous spread occurs when the microorganism source is from other people or the environment [1, 8, 9].

Risk Factors

The risk factors for HAIs vary between the different healthcare contexts. For acute care the common risks are age (65 years or older); emergency admission; admission to ICU; insertion of a central venous line, indwelling catheter or respiratory intubation; surgical intervention; and immunosuppressed state [1, 9]. In residential care facilities several factors increase the likelihood of HAIs. Firstly the age profile of residents makes this cohort vulnerable, with studies demonstrating that the elderly are generally at higher risk of pneumonia and urinary tract infections. Group living poses a significant risk factor as well. In addition the presence of feeding tubes, urinary catheters, and pressure areas caused by immobility put these residents at risk [8].

Common HAIs

The common HAIs are related to the risk factors identified above, with infections linked to urinary catheters, surgical sites, ventilator associated pneumonia, and the use of intravascular devices accounting for 80 per cent of all HAIs [10]. Other HAIs which occur less frequently than the 'top four' but are nevertheless not uncommon are related to soft tissue injury and subsequent infection such as pressure ulcers and burns, enteric infections and respiratory infections [11]. The evidence is clear that if health professionals comply with infection prevention strategies (especially hand hygiene) the prevalence of HAIs is reduced significantly [1, 5–7, 12–17]. Attention to hand cleansing protocols is the most common strategy and easiest to institute. Hand hygiene and other general strategies will be discussed later in the chapter, but first we will look briefly at the common HAIs and specific prevention strategies associated with them.

Infections related to urinary catheters

Urinary tract infections account for 36 per cent of all HAIs, with the majority (80 per cent) of urinary tract infections linked to urinary catheters [18]. The risk factors for these infections include the length of time the urinary catheter is in place, patient age and history of malignancy [2]. These infections have a lower mortality and morbidity than other HAIs, but they increase the financial cost of care and the discomfort of patients considerably [1, 2]. Prevention strategies are a strict adherence to aseptic insertion technique (see information on bundles below), maintaining a closed drainage system, avoiding the use of a catheter unless absolutely clinically required, removal of catheter as soon as clinically possible, and appropriate catheter care [11].

Surgical site infections

Surgical site infections comprise approximately 20 per cent of all HAIs [18]. The risks of a surgical site infection are increased if the surgery is related to trauma, if the surgery is prolonged or if the patient has medical comorbidities [2, 11]. Prevention strategies include the practice of optimal surgical technique, maintenance of clean environment, sterile equipment, appropriate use of prophylactic antibiotics, and using clippers rather than razors for pre-op hair removal [2, 11].

Pneumonias related to ventilators

Pneumonias related to ventilators (VAPs) account for 11 per cent of all HAIs and have the highest mortality. About 15 per cent of patients who are ventilated will get a VAP, and VAP is the most common HAI in ICUs [2, 16]. However, similarly to other HAIs, compliance with VAP prevention strategies significantly impacts on reducing the rate [12, 16]. These strategies include nursing the patient in a semi-recumbent position with the head of the bed elevated to at least 30 degrees. Oral care including brushing teeth, rinsing the mouth, oral suctioning and attention to the storing, rinsing and replacement of suctioning equipment has been shown in some studies to reduce the incidence of VAP. However, oral care protocols are not universally utilised in ICUs so this area requires some consideration [16]. The duration of intubation increases the likelihood of VAP, so weaning from the ventilator and removal of the tube as soon as clinically possible is an important strategy. The VAP bundle (see more general information on bundles below) includes nursing the patient in a semi-recumbent position (as noted above) and also a daily interruption of sedation and deep vein thrombosis and peptic ulcer prophylaxis. Adherence to the VAP bundles shows a reduction in VAPs of 45 per cent [16].

Intravascular device infections

Localised skin infections and bloodstream HAIs can occur with the use of an intravascular device (IVD), with IVD bloodstream HAIs accounting for 11 per cent of all HAIs [18]. The principal strategy for the prevention of HAIs related to IVDs is to avoid using them unless there is a compelling clinical indication and to remove them as soon as clinically possible. Ensuring strict asepsis on insertion, maintenance and removal, and evidence based care of the IVD site, is also a key reduction strategy [13, 14]. IVD care bundles (see below) incorporating these features have also been developed. There is strong evidence that these care bundles have a marked effect on the reduction of HAIs related to IVD; studies focusing on central line-associated infections demonstrate a 66 per cent reduction [13, 14].

Prevention of HAIs

Many of the HAI prevention strategies require changes and implementation at an organisational level. These organisational strategies include the introduction of an infection control and surveillance programme, planning for building and reconstruction of buildings, food safety and waste management programmes, adequate disinfection and sterilisation of surgical instruments and endoscopic equipment, compliance with antimicrobial guidelines, and the development of policies and procedures to manage clinical and environmental infection control risks. However, in this chapter we will focus on strategies for which individual practitioners can be responsible and accountable.

In the previous sections we mentioned bundles of care in relation to the four most common HAIs. Bundles of care provide a good starting point for a discussion about prevention. We will then briefly discuss standard precautions in relation to the prevention of infection, and from there move on to the most important strategy for the reduction of infections – hand hygiene.

Bundles of care

In Chapter 1 we noted that humans are prone to making mistakes, slips and errors as a result of the way we process information and work at tasks using conscious and automatic processing. Utilising this knowledge the discipline of human factors focuses on developing workplace strategies to lessen the likelihood that errors will occur. Bundles of care are one such strategy. Recognising humans' susceptibility to omit steps in a process or to carry the steps out but in the wrong order led to the development of care bundles. These care bundles are a set of evidence based practices that are mandatory in the undertaking of a particular task.

The steps (there should be no more than four or five for maximum effectiveness) are based on random control trials (RCTs) with robust levels of evidence (levels 1 and 2). The steps involved are accepted and well-established practice in themselves but as part of the care bundle they must be performed together every time for the intervention they are designed for. The difference between a bundle and a checklist is that a bundle contains small but critical processes all determined by level 1 or 2 evidence, whereas a checklist contains 'nice to do' tasks as well as 'mandatory' tasks and normally lists a number of steps. Some examples of bundles are the central vascular catheter (CVC) bundle, peripheral vascular catheter (PVC) bundle and catheter associated urinary tract infections (CAUTI) bundle. When adopted by an organisation it has been demonstrated that there are significant reductions in the HAIs associated with these processes [17].

Standard precautions

Standard precautions are practices that should be used for all patients at all times. They include assessing the need for, and then using if required, gloves, masks, eye protection and gowns for different procedures and care provision. They also incorporate effective cleaning and maintenance of equipment (think of the common things like blood pressure cuffs, temperature probes, and pulse oximetry equipment) as well as proper handling and disposal of sharps. The consideration of patient placement dependent on the level of risk is also part of the suite of standard precautions [9, 11]. Finally, and most importantly, is attention to hand hygiene, which is considered to be the principal standard precaution.

Hand hygiene

Hand hygiene has become the single most important method of preventing HAIs [8, 9, 18, 19]. While patients, their families and other visitors may be the transmission agent, it is clear that the hands of healthcare workers are a significant cause of both endogenous and exogenous transmission. Given that hand hygiene is a basic precaution routinely advocated since the 1800s when Dr Semmelweis demonstrated that washing hands reduced childbirth related infections from 10 to 1 per cent [20] it is hard to understand why compliance rates by healthcare workers have been and remain low, with studies reporting rates as low as 20–50 per cent compliance [4, 20, 21] both in developed and developing countries. The World Health Organization has recognised the quantum of the problem and the challenges involved in addressing it, and in 2009 launched the *SAVE LIVES: Clean Your Hands* campaign (www.who.int/gpsc/ 5may/background/en/). This campaign aims to improve hand hygiene across the world in all healthcare contexts. The key point of the campaign identifies the 'five moments' in the clinical setting when it is imperative that hand hygiene occurs. They are:

• before touching a patient
• before clean/aseptic procedure
• after body fluid exposure risk
• after touching a patient, and
• after touching patient surrounds [18].

Wearing gloves does not absolve the health professional from the need for hand hygiene – if at any of the 'five moments' gloves are worn then following the intervention they must be removed and hand hygiene completed [18].

However, the key to effective hand hygiene is not only cleaning hands at those five moments but also cleaning them adequately with either an alcohol-based hand rub or soap and water. The technique for each, while not difficult, is important. The following exercise targets each of the techniques.

Exercise 3.1

Aim of the exercise: To identify the principal elements of the technique for both hand rub and hand washing with soap and water.

What to do:

1. Go to the WHO website for hand hygiene: www.who.int/gpsc/ 5may/Hand_Hygiene_Why_How_and_When_Brochure.pdf.
2. Review this brochure and write down the key points for the techniques for hand rub and hand washing.
3. Using this information, review your own technique for each of these. It may help to practise using the posters as a guide. How good was your technique before you reviewed this information? Identify the specific changes you have had to make to your technique.

4. Discuss your findings with colleagues or friends. You may like to demonstrate the correct technique for hand rubs and hand washing and ask them for their feedback about their own practice.
5. Compare your findings with the Exercise Feedback section at the end of the chapter.

Hand hygiene seems such a simple process yet its impact on reduction of HAIs is remarkable. What then are the barriers to health professionals completing this simple task each time they should? The factors cited in different studies include a lack of time and busyness of the workload, lack of knowledge of the importance of hand hygiene, lack of role models from colleagues and other health professionals, forgetting to undertake hand hygiene when moving from task to task, and a lack of organisational support [2, 4, 7–9, 18–21]. The following story illustrates some of these barriers.

Sinéad's story

Sinéad (24) worked in a very busy paediatric surgical ward in a major teaching hospital. The work environment was challenging but the team as a whole was very supportive and highly motivated. It was the type of setting that a young, ambitious and hard working professional could thrive in. It suited Sinéad to a tee. It was her first day back at work after a week of sand and surf in Queensland and she was looking forward to catching up with colleagues and friends. She started back on an afternoon shift but the ward was nothing short of 'chaotic' compared with the usual smooth running machine it normally was. A common flu had confined several senior and regular staff to bed and the replacements were unable to cope effectively with the workload. Being familiar with the setting Sinéad rolled up her sleeves and started to work after a brief handover. About 80 minutes later she went to attend to one of the patients in her care – a two-year-old who had undergone a surgical procedure to remove tonsils and adenoids earlier that morning. As Sinéad approached the bedside with a smile the mother of the child, who was also a nurse, asked 'Nurse, have you washed your hands?' The question stopped Sinéad in her tracks. She knew that in the short time that she was at work her failure to follow a simple hand-washing protocol consistently had potentially undermined people's care and placed them at risk.

With our knowledge of human factors, a number of strategies can be used to address these barriers to improve compliance with hand hygiene. Firstly, it should be ensured that resources such as hand rub and handbasins are placed where staff have easy access to them – for example hand rub situated at bedsides and entry to patients' rooms, and handbasins situated close to all clinical activity. Where this may involve a large capital cost, simply providing individual healthcare professionals with their own pocket hand rub may be an economical solution. These strategies tackle the human propensity to forget to do tasks when distracted or busy (slips and lapses), and decrease the likelihood of violations related to a lack of resources. Other strategies involve education and training programmes to raise the level of awareness of the impact of hand hygiene on HAIs.

Exercise 3.2

Aim of the exercise: To identify the actions you can take as a health professional that make a significant difference to the likelihood of a patient acquiring an HAI.

What to do:

1. Review the contents of this chapter as well as some of the following websites:

   • www.nhmrc.gov.au/_files_nhmrc/publications/attachments/cd33_infection_control_healthcare_0.pdf
   • www.chp.gov.hk/files/pdf/guideline_prevention_of_communicable_diseases_rchd_4_infection_control_measures.pdf
   • www.who.int/csr/resources/publications/drugresist/en/whocdscsreph200212.pdf
   • www.who.int/csr/resources/publications/EPR_AM2_E7.pdf.

2. Now make a list of those things you can do as an individual health professional that will contribute to the prevention of HAIs.
3. Discuss your findings with colleagues or friends.
4. Compare your findings with the Exercise Feedback section at the end of the chapter.

Summary

In this chapter we have provided a brief background to HAIs, a very significant problem for the healthcare system and a major impediment to quality outcomes for patients. We have reviewed the evidence based strategies that should be common practice to prevent or minimise HAIs. However, it is evident that, even though these strategies are relatively simple, adherence to them by healthcare workers is not high. The take home message from this chapter is that *The Little Things Count*. The simplicity of interventions versus the cost saving in dollars and in human impact seems not to attract the excitement and attention that focuses the resources and support that result in major changes to improve outcomes for patients. Until this happens there will be little impact on the incidence rates of HAIs.

In the next chapter we will review another type of common adverse event – those that occur as a result of medication errors.

The themes of this chapter relate to the WHO curriculum guideline topics of [10]:

- Why human factors are important in patient safety
- Infection prevention and control.

The Exercise Feedback below provides an overview of the key points of this chapter.

EXERCISE FEEDBACK

Exercise 3.1

The posters available at the site you were directed to for this exercise (www.who.int/gpsc/5may/Hand_Hygiene_Why_How_and_When_Brochure. pdf) provide excellent illustrations of the two techniques. However, the summary below is provided for completeness.

The essential elements for hand rub involve:

- duration of procedure 20–30 seconds
- applying product to cupped hand
- rubbing hands palm to palm
- rubbing right hand over left dorsum with interlaced fingers and vice versa

- rubbing palm to palm with interlaced fingers
- rubbing backs of fingers to opposing palms with fingers interlocked
- rotational rubbing of left thumb clasped in right palm and vice versa
- rotational rubbing, backwards and forwards with clasped fingers of right hand in left palm and vice versa
- once dry, hand hygiene is complete.
- The essential elements for hand washing involve:
- duration of procedure 40–60 seconds
- wet hands with water
- apply soap to cover all hand surfaces
- rub hands palm to palm
- rubbing right hand over left dorsum with interlaced fingers and vice versa
- rubbing palm to palm with interlaced fingers
- rubbing backs of fingers to opposing palms with fingers interlocked
- rotational rubbing of left thumb clasped in right palm and vice versa
- rotational rubbing, backwards and forwards with clasped fingers of right hand in left palm and vice versa
- rinse hands with water
- dry hands thoroughly with a single use towel
- use towel to turn off tap – hand hygiene is complete.

The key of course is to undertake hand hygiene for each of the five moments using the above techniques.

Exercise 3.2

The key elements of effective practice by an individual practitioner to reduce HAIs are:

- the consistent practice and promotion of hand hygiene
- familiarity with, assessment of the requirement for, and the use of standard precautions for every patient
- for prevention of catheter related urinary tract infections – strict adherence to aseptic insertion technique, maintaining a closed drainage system, avoiding the use of a catheter unless absolutely clinically required, removal of catheter as soon as clinically possible, and appropriate catheter care
- for prevention of surgical site infections – the practice of optimal surgical technique, maintenance of clean environment, sterile equipment,

appropriate use of prophylactic antibiotics, and using clippers rather than razors for pre-op hair removal

- for prevention of VAPs – nursing the patient in a semi-recumbent position with the head of the bed elevated to at least 30 degrees, oral care, extubation as soon as clinically possible, and daily interruption of sedation and deep vein thrombosis and peptic ulcer prophylaxis
- for prevention of infections related to IVDs – ensuring strict asepsis on insertion, maintenance and removal of the IVDs, evidence based care of the IVD site, and removal as soon as clinically indicated
- the use of bundles of care where they are part of organisational policy and procedure; where they are not part of organisational policy and procedure, the promotion of these as an effective strategy to decrease HAIs.

HAIs are a significant issue for patient safety but you as an individual practitioner can have a significant impact on reducing their occurrence.

References

1. *Report on the Burden of Endemic Health Care Associated Infection*, 2011, Geneva: World Health Organization.
2. Wachter, R., *Understanding Patient Safety*. 2nd ed. 2012, San Francisco: McGraw-Hill.
3. *Private and Public Hospitals: Research report*, 2009, Canberra: Productivity Commission.
4. Barrett, R. and J. Randle, *Hand hygiene practices: Nursing students' perceptions*. Journal of Clinical Nursing, 2008. **17**(14): 1851–1857.
5. Hassan, M., et al., *Cost of hospital acquired infection*. Hospital Topics, 2010. **88**(3): 82–89.
6. Allegranzi, B., et al., *Burden of endemic healthcare associated infection in developing countries: Systematic review and meta-analysis*. Lancet, 2011. **377**: 228–241.
7. Allegranzi, B., et al., *Successful implementation of the World Health Organization hand hygiene improvement strategy in a referral hospital in Mali, Africa*. Infection Control Hospital Epidemiology, 2010. **31**(2): 133–141.
8. *Hand Hygiene in Outpatient and Home-based and Long-term Care Facilities*, 2012, Geneva: World Health Organization.
9. Curtis, L., *Prevention of hospital-acquired infections: Review of non-pharmalogical interventions*. Journal of Hospital Infection, 2008. **69**: 204–219.
10. *WHO Patient Safety Curriculum Guide: Multi-professional edition*, 2011, Geneva: World Health Organization.
11. *Prevention of Hospital Acquired Infections: A practical guide*, 2002, Geneva: World Health Organization.

12. De Palo, V., et al., *The Rhode Island Collaborative: A model for reducing central line-associated bloodstream infection and ventilator-assisted pneumonia statewide.* Quality and Safety in Health Care, 2010. **19**: 555–561.

13. Pronovost, P., et al., *Sustaining reductions in catheter related bloodstream infections in Michigan intensive care units: Observational study.* BMJ, 2010. **340**: c309.

14. Pronovost, P., et al., *An intervention to decrease catheter-related bloodstream infections in the ICU.* New England Journal of Medicine, 2006. **355**: 2725–2732.

15. Fulbrook, P. and S. Mooney, *Care bundles in critical care: A practical approach to evidence based practice.* British Association of Critical Care Nursing in Critical Care, 2003. **8**(6): 249–255.

16. Ruffell, A. and L. Adamcova, *Ventilator-associated pneumonia: Prevention is better than cure.* British Association of Critical Care Nursing in Critical Care, 2008. **13**(1): 44–53.

17. Robb, E., et al., *Using care bundles to reduce in-hospital mortality: Quantitative survey.* BMJ, 2010. **340**: c1234.

18. *WHO Guidelines on Hand Hygiene in Health Care,* 2009, Geneva: World Health Organization.

19. *Guide to the Implementation of the WHO Multimodal Hand Hygiene Improvement Strategy,* 2009, Geneva: World Health Organization.

20. Creedon, S., *Heathcare workers' hand decontamination practices: Compliance with recommended guidelines.* Journal of Advanced Nursing, 2005. **51**: 208–216.

21. Pittet, D., *Improving adherence to hand hygiene practice: A multidisciplinary approach.* Emerging Infectious Diseases, 2001. **7**(2): 235–240.

4

Medication Errors

Introduction

The case study above is a profound reminder of the dire consequences that can result from a medication error. One can imagine how easy it is to make this sort of terrible error in an emergency situation, when there are heightened stress levels – especially with our knowledge that when processing information humans are prone to errors. Unfortunately medication errors are one of the most common adverse events reported; fortunately most do not result in the type of catastrophic outcome reported in the case study above, but many do result in harm to patients [1, 2]. The different types of medication errors include prescribing, dispensing, preparation and administration errors [3]. Patients can experience these errors at any stage of the healthcare encounter, with approximately 3 per cent from prescribing and around 19 per cent in administration. Errors in preadmission documentation of medication history occur around 20 per cent of the time, and about 25 per cent of patients will have errors in their discharge prescriptions [2, 4–6]. Medication errors are not limited to the hospital setting – approximately 1 in 20 hospital admissions are related to medication prescribed in the community setting, and those in residential homecare settings have also been shown to be at risk from medication administration errors [7, 8]. Many factors can lead to a medication error, some of which are organisational and others human. Understanding the factors contributing to medication errors allows us to identify strategies that will reduce the likelihood of an error occurring.

In this chapter we will review the different types of medication errors and then move on to examine the factors that can contribute to them. Finally we will consider strategies that organisations and individual clinicians can implement to reduce their likelihood. We will begin, though, by defining what we mean by medication errors.

Defining Medication Errors

When we talk about medication errors it is important to be explicit about what we are and are not including. There is some disagreement about the definition of a medication error [9] – for instance do we include 'near misses', where the error was detected and stopped before it reached the patient? What about errors where the patient suffered no harm, or errors that occur in the dispensing of the medication rather than the administration? Of course, in any discussion or study of medication errors it is essential that we are talking about the same thing and comparing 'apples with apples'. So for the purposes of this chapter we will be using the very comprehensive definition from the National Coordinating Council for Medication Error Reporting and Prevention (2005):

> A medication error is any preventable event that may cause or lead to inappropriate medication use or patient harm while the medication is in the control of the health care professional, patient, or

consumer. Such events may be related to professional practice, health care products, procedures, and systems, including prescribing; order communication; product labeling, packaging, and nomenclature; compounding; dispensing; distribution; administration; education; monitoring; and use. [9]

Types of Medication Errors

Medication errors can occur at all stages of the process including prescription, dispensing and administration. This is an important point to make, as often the focus is on the administration stage (where most errors are reported) [1, 2], which involves principally nurses. However, errors do occur at the other stages and these can involve doctors, pharmacists, clerical staff and other support staff [10]. Thus, medication error causation and therefore prevention must be viewed as multidisciplinary. We will now look at each stage separately.

Prescription errors

Prescription errors can involve prescribing the wrong drug for a patient or prescribing the wrong dose and/or quantity of the drug. It may be that several drugs are prescribed for the patient and there is an interaction between the drugs, or the patient has a known allergy to the drug – these are classed as adverse drug reactions. By far the most common cause of prescribing errors, however, is related to the use of abbreviations and drug expressions, and poor handwriting [9, 11]. There are several good practice principles that should be followed when prescribing medication (see Table 4.1). These principles are adapted from the Australian Commission on Safety and Quality in Healthcare medication policy document [9], but other countries have similar guidelines.

The principles are pretty straightforward, yet there is a strong history of the use of Latin terms and for practitioners not to write legibly and clearly because they are too busy, or to use symbols to communicate with other 'experts'. Whatever the reason or reasons, it is dangerous and we must seek to change these patterns of behaviour. Have you ever considered why these unsafe patterns of prescribing persist?

Table 4.1   Good practice principles when prescribing medication

1	Use plain English – no jargon
2	Write in full – avoid using abbreviations wherever possible, including Latin abbreviations
3	Print all text – especially drug names
4	Use generic drug names
5	Write drug name in full. Never abbreviate any drug name
6	Do not use chemical symbols
7	Use words or numbers – not Roman numerals
	Use metric units – not apothecary units
	Use a leading zero in front of a decimal point for a dose less than 1 and do not use trailing zeros after a decimal point
	For oral liquid preparations express dose in weight as well as volume
	Express dosage frequency unambiguously
8	Do not use fractions
9	Do not use symbols
10	Avoid acronyms or abbreviations for medical terms and procedures on orders or prescriptions

Adapted from *Recommendations for Terminology, Abbreviations and Symbols used in the Prescribing and Administration of Medicines* (2010) [9]. Reprinted with permission from Australian Commission on Safety and Quality in Healthcare.

Exercise 4.1

Aim of the exercise: To explore your ideas about why professionals do not follow good practice principles for medication prescriptions.

What to do:

1. Read the following statements and make some notes to summarise your own views on these:

   - Using abbreviations and jargon helps busy practitioners to communicate effectively and efficiently.
   - Most people assume that others can read their handwriting.
   - If people don't understand a medication order they can ask the prescriber about it.
   - Being a professional means communicating in specialised ways.
   - Most patients don't want to know details about the medication they are prescribed so handwriting is not important.

2. After you have noted down some ideas share your thoughts and opinions on these with others informally. What stands out in the

conversation that might shed some light on our understanding about the continued use of jargon in spite of the good practice guidelines highlighted in Table 4.1?

3. Compare your findings with the Exercise Feedback section at the end of the chapter.

Dispensing errors

Dispensing errors occur when the drug dispensed differs from the drug prescribed. This results when the order is misinterpreted either in terms of the drug itself, the dose of the drug or the quantity of the drug. Other errors that can occur in the dispensing are if the label is generated incorrectly and/or affixed to the wrong package or container. The final process of dispensing where there is a possibility of error relates to ensuring that the prescription is given to the correct patient [9].

Medication dispensing case studies

A pharmacist dispensed the antihypertensive felodipine (Plendil®) 20 mg four times a day having misread a prescription for 'Isordil®', used to treat angina, 20 mg four times a day. The patient died following a cardiac arrest.

A man suffered irreversible brain damage after a pharmacist misread his doctor's prescription. The patient had been prescribed the antibiotic Amoxil® (amoxicillin) for a chest infection. The prescription was badly written and the pharmacist misread the drug name as Daonil® (glibenclamide), a drug used to lower blood sugar in people with diabetes. As a result of taking the wrong medicine the patient went into a coma and was hospitalised for five months. He suffered blunted intellect and poor short-term memory as a direct result of the medication error.

The dispensing errors in the case studies above may have been the result of the pharmacist having to interpret poor handwriting or the medications being in similar packages and stored close together. The use of trade names versus the recommended use of generic names may have contributed to the second incident. The organisational factors that may lead to these errors are discussed later in the chapter.

Administration errors

Clinicians have been traditionally taught the 'five rights' of medication administration [8]. These are:

- right patient
- right drug
- right route
- right time
- right dose.

An administration error occurs when any one of these 'rights' is breached. The administration of medication is where the majority of errors occur as there are multiple steps in this process that can go wrong. Wrong dose, dose omission, and wrong administration time are the most common administration error types. As with dispensing errors, frequent causes of administration errors are orders in which the drug name, dose or route are illegible (see case study below). This problem can occur because of poor handwriting of the prescriber, but also because some letters, numerals, abbreviations and dose designations can be easily confused. Table 4.2 provides examples. Misheard verbal orders and transcription mistakes of medication orders can also lead to errors [6].

Table 4.2 Examples of letters, numerals, abbreviations and dose designations that can be easily confused [12–14]

Lower case l and	Upper case I
Lower case o and	Numeral 0
Lower case c and	Lower case e
Upper case S and	Numeral 5
Numeral 3 and	Numeral 8
IN (intranasal) mistaken as	IM (intramuscular)
mcg (micrograms) mistaken as	mg (milligrams)
SC (subcutaneous) mistaken as	SL (sublingual)
SS (sliding scale) mistaken as	55
6/24 (every 6 hours) mistaken as	6 times a day
1.0 mg mistaken as	10 mg (if decimal point not seen)
.5 mg mistaken as	5 mg (if decimal point not seen)
K (potassium) mistaken as	Vit K
@ (at) mistaken as	2

Medication administration case study

A 15-year-old boy with end-stage AIDS was admitted to the paediatric ICU with mental status changes. He was diagnosed with status epilepticus and started on a loading dose of IV phenytoin.

In the step-down unit, the resident wrote an order for a maintenance dose of phenytoin. The order was written as mg/kg/d without specification that 'd' meant day not dose. As a result, the patient received approximately three times the indicated dose. Later that day, a pharmacist called to alert the resident to his mistake. The subsequent phenytoin level was 98 (therapeutic range 10–20).

Reprinted with permission of AHRQ WebM&M. Source: Kaushal R. Medication overdose. AHRQ WebM&M [serial online]. April 2003. Available at: www.webmm.ahrq.gov/case.aspx?caseID=9.

The case above provides a clear example of the type of error that can occur when there is a misunderstanding on the part of the health professional about the dose of medication. In this case the one of the 'five rights' that was breached was the right dose. This error could have been avoided if the best practice guidelines of not using abbreviations had been followed.

Most medications are available in the dosage that is usually prescribed. However, there are still occasions when clinicians are required to calculate the dosage, volume or rate of the medication required for the particular patient. At times these calculations can be complex, and may require working from dilution (1 in 1000) to concentration (1 mg per ml) and ratio (0.1 per cent). The risk of error is high, especially when the calculation is being carried out in stressful and time critical situations. This was well illustrated in a study reported in 2008 where doctors were required to calculate the correct dose of epinephrine (also known as adrenaline and used to treat allergic reactions or heart attacks) in a simulated emergency situation. Epinephrine can be presented as a dose (1 mg per ml) or a ratio (1:1000). Doctors who had to calculate the dosage when the drug was presented as a ratio took 1.5 times longer than those who were presented with it as a dosage, and all but two out of 28 doctors overdosed the simulated patient [15].

Another risk at the administration stage is when the clinician is selecting the drug for administration and look-alike or sound-alike drug names or similar packaging cause confusion [14]. These are selection

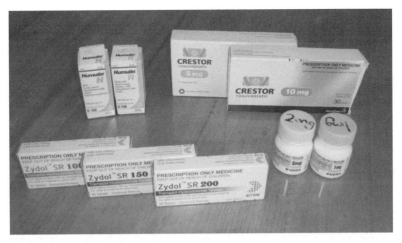

Figure 4.1   Examples of different dosages of medication in similar packages

errors as explained in human factors theory. The case study presented at the beginning of this chapter is an example. This can also happen when different dosages of the same drug are presented in similar packaging. Figure 4.1 shows an example of similar packaging of different dosages of medication.

It is clear that the process of medication prescribing, dispensing and administering is fraught with possible danger for patients, and a source of potential errors in care for all of the multidisciplinary team involved. We will now move on to discuss the factors that contribute to medication errors.

Factors that Contribute to Medication Errors

In Chapter 1 we discussed some of the factors that increase the likelihood of errors occurring. We identified that latent factors leading to errors were those where organisational systems, which should be in place to prevent errors, fail. Human factors that lead to errors at the clinician/patient interface are labelled active errors. Both latent and human factors can be linked specifically to medication errors. There is an intricate relationship between organisational/system factors (latent errors) and human factors (active errors) which, in the case of a medication error, makes it impossible to completely separate any one factor as the causative one (think back to Chapter 1 and the Swiss

Cheese model of error). However, while recognising the interconnectedness of organisational/system and human factors that lead to medication errors, we will deal with each separately in the following discussion.

Organisational factors that lead to medication errors

There is a clear relationship in the literature between work environment factors and the likelihood of medication errors [15]. Heavy workloads, rapidly changing situations (acute care, emergency situations, frequent changes of orders and care plans, high numbers of admissions and discharges), staff shortages and staff working in unfamiliar clinical contexts all lead to situations in which clinicians are frequently interrupted and subject to multiple distractions.

We have established that medication administration is a complex process, thus it follows that anyone taking part in the process who is distracted or interrupted is more likely to make mistakes [16]. An example of this is the hypothetical situation where a nurse administering oral Lasix (a medication which increases urine output) to a patient realises that the patient may need a potassium supplement as well. On the way to check the patient's electrolyte results she is interrupted by another nurse and then by a relative. After finishing both conversations she returns to the medication round completely forgetting to check the patient's requirement for potassium.

Team factors such as the quality of communication and teamwork between the different professionals also interface with the likelihood of medication errors [17]. Where there is good communication and teamwork there is increased likelihood that nurses and other clinicians will question and investigate medication orders. Conversely, poor communication and inadequate handover between clinicians is more likely to lead to errors.

Medication packaging, handling, storage and delivery systems are important considerations for medication safety. As mentioned above, medication packaging that is similar increases the chances of error, and storing medications with similar packaging and/or similar names in close proximity to each other can lead to inadvertent mix-ups when a busy nurse, pharmacist or doctor is reaching for a particular medication [18]. As well, medication systems that do not meet the requirements for timely administration of the drugs to patients will lead clinicians to develop workaround systems such as using another patient's medication while waiting for medication to arrive [19].

Human factors that lead to medication errors

In Chapter 1 we identified that human factors involves the study of the relationship between human beings and the systems they interact with, and uses this knowledge to design strategies to optimise human performance [20]. We discussed how humans undertake actions either consciously with focused attention or automatically with little conscious thought. The automatic behaviour, which all humans utilise to function effectively, allows us to multi-task. However, this normal human behaviour also has a downside in that it makes us more likely to make an unintentional error. These errors are classified as slips, lapses and mistakes [21]. This general understanding about the likelihood of slips, lapses and mistakes can be applied specifically to medication errors.

Slips and lapses can be related to misidentification of objects or messages. These occur as we see or hear what we expect to see or hear. This may be as a result of inattentional blindness [18, 21]. For example, if we are used to seeing a particular medication in a particular coloured package then when we are presented with a different medication with very similar packaging we are likely not to recognise that it is a different medication. An illustration of this was a situation where an experienced nurse was drawing up the drugs during a resuscitation and inadvertently drew up calcium chloride instead of adrenaline as the drugs were stored in similar boxes next to each other in the resuscitation area. The only difference was that the calcium chloride box had a yellow stripe and the adrenaline had a grey stripe down the side of the box. Fortunately this did not alter the outcome for the patient.

Here is a simple example of how we perceive things in line with our view of the world. If you ask people to describe what they see when they look at Figure 4.2 many of them will say a pig's or an elephant's rump. Why? The reason is that our brains are designed to fill in the missing bits and to give things meaning in accord with our experience and expectations [22]. However, the figure is made up of some shapes located in a particular order – nothing more.

This example highlights the ease with which a person can fill in missing bits of information and see things that are not there, or see them differently, potentially leading to a serious mistake.

Slips and lapses can also occur when we are distracted or interrupted while in the middle of doing something [21]. An example of this might be when you start to get organised to give a patient their morning insulin and are interrupted by other requests from patients which

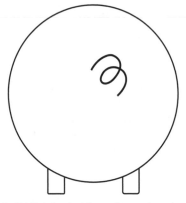

Figure 4.2   What is this? Adapted from Ramachandran (2011) [22]. Used by permission of W.W. Norton and Company, Inc.

occupy some of your time. You then go on to deal with other tasks and duties and only realise you have not given the insulin when the patient experiences a hyperglycaemic event.

Similarly, consider an example where you have administered a patient's IM analgesia but before you get a chance to sign the medication chart indicating the time and dose the patient becomes nauseous and vomits all over themselves and their bed-linen. By the time you have finished assisting the patient and settling them down comfortably you have forgotten that the chart has not been signed. You only remember at handover when you note that another nurse gave the patient more analgesia an hour later.

Mistakes occur when we apply a solution to a situation based on a solution that has worked before. An example of this type of error applied to medication is when a patient has been ordered Heparin 500 units, the nurse who is caring for the patient knows that the dose used for patients to prevent blood clots is Heparin 5000 units, and misreads the prescription as Heparin 5000 units and therefore draws up Heparin 5000 units and administers this to flush the IV line. However, the dose for flushing IV lines is 500 units.

So slips, lapses and mistakes can lead to unintentional medication errors. Violations, however, are intentional behaviours that an individual chooses to carry out because the resources are not available or it is difficult or impossible to apply the rule. If we relate this specifically to medication errors, an example of a violation that may occur if resources are not available is if a patient is ordered a particular medication but there is a long delay in the medication arriving on the ward. In this situation it is not uncommon for a nurse to choose to use another patient's medication that is available on the ward. The likelihood of the wrong dose, the wrong drug or drug allergy going undetected is increased when there is a workaround like this, as the checks that are undertaken when a pharmacist dispenses a medication to a particular patient are missed out of the process [12].

An example of a violation that may occur if it is difficult to apply the rule is a situation where the policy on medication administration requires that a second checker is used to confirm the 'five rights' of correct dose, person, time, medication and route. However, because of staff shortages there is no one available on the ward and so rather than calling for someone from another area, and waiting a considerable time for the second checker to arrive, the nurse may choose to ignore the policy and give the medication without the second check. In a 'once off' situation the nurse may be so aware of the possibility of error because there is a deviation from the policy that the conscious focus lessens the likelihood of error. However, if this situation occurs regularly the violation becomes more routine and likelihood of an error increases [23].

So, having discussed some of the key organisational and human factors that increase the chances of a medication error we will now examine some strategies that help prevent such errors. However, before we do this, complete the following exercise.

Exercise 4.2

Aim of the exercise: To identify the organisational/system and human factors that contribute to system errors.

What to do:

1. Read the following case study:

   An 87-year-old man was 5 days postoperative from a decompressive laminectomy (an orthopaedic spinal operation). Although he suffered from dementia, he remained alert and oriented with only mild short-term memory loss. During his stay at a rehabilitation unit, a nursing student administered a 'cup' of medications that included clopidogrel (Plavix), carbidopa-levodopa (Sinemet), prednisone, rivastigmine tartrate (Exelon), and risperidone (Risperdal). Unfortunately, this cup of medications belonged to another patient on the unit. As a result, the patient became drowsy with mild nausea and hypotension, but the symptoms resolved within 24 hours without further event. After learning about the error, the family requested no further care from any nursing students.

On this particular unit, nursing students receive supervision from a senior nursing instructor. The unit's policy required that only the instructors access Pyxis (an automated drug dispensing system) when administering medications. In this case, the instructor attempted to save time by having the eight nursing students prepare their medications from Pyxis at the same time; after preparation, the instructor reviewed each student's understanding of the medication(s) and preparation accuracy. After this process was completed, the students left each of their patients' medication(s) in a 'cup' on the counter in the medication room. When the time came to administer the medication(s), the student in this case picked up the wrong cup of medications for her patient.

The error was discovered when a different student expecting to give the above medications reviewed the ones in her cup and discovered the wrong medications – also a near miss for her patient.

Reprinted with permission of AHRQ WebM&M. Source: Blegen MA, Pepper GA. Cups of error. AHRQ WebM&M [serial online]. May 2006. Available at: www.webmm.ahrq.gov/case.aspx?caseID=125.

2. Now make a note of the organisation/system factors and the human factors that may have contributed to this error.
3. Discuss your findings with friends/colleagues.
4. In your discussions also identify any strategies that you think may help prevent situations like this happening again in the future.
5. After you have read the next section of this chapter, return to this exercise and note down if you can add any further prevention strategies to your findings.
6. Compare your findings with the Exercise Feedback section at the end of the chapter.

Strategies to Decrease Medication Errors

We have identified previously that the process of prescribing, dispensing and administering medication involves many systems and processes and several different professions. At any stage in the process either something can go wrong with the systems that support it or human factors can disorder it. Therefore any strategies to decrease the likelihood of errors must be targeted at both the organisational/system factors and the human factors that lead to errors.

Human factors

In the previous section we looked at the influence of human factors on the possibility of errors. Many of the environmental, equipment and workplace strategies to reduce medication errors have been developed based on our knowledge of human factors. Modifying or managing the working conditions which are more likely to produce errors – such as short staffing, frequent changes of orders, interruptions during medication rounds, multiple admissions and discharges, and lack of supervision – is a positive move towards minimising the likelihood of a medication error. In some clinical areas staff wear an identifying vest when preparing or administering medication indicating that they must not be interrupted. Other staff and patients are educated that they must not interrupt or distract nurses wearing these vests [8]. In one hospital this tactic was shown to reduce medication errors by 20 per cent [12].

Protocols that call for double-checking of the 'five rights' during medication dispensing and administration are another strategy for minimising risk of errors [16]. However, it is critical that these checks are seen as an important part of the process rather than as a rubber-stamping. It is also important to include those involved in the checking process in the development of the protocols to ensure they are practical in the clinical setting.

Our knowledge of human factors – the predisposition to making mistakes, slips, lapses and violations which are exacerbated by stress, distraction and poorly designed workplaces – provides us with the opportunity to develop specific strategies involving the prescribing, dispensing and administration of medications to prevent errors. The following sections detail some of these strategies for minimising medication errors such as recognising and addressing organisational culture, standardising terms, computerised systems, the storage and packaging of medications, involvement of pharmacists, and including patients in care.

Organisational culture

Poor organisational structures and processes and human factors are aggravated in organisations where there is a culture that tolerates risky behaviour. The healthcare practitioners in such organisations generally do not recognise that the accepted practices pose extra risks to patients, however, as it is just 'how things are done around here'. In these organisations the systems to monitor and support good practice in patient safety tend to be inadequate, and there is often poor communication and ineffective teamwork [24]. Positive safety cultures demonstrate a commitment to systems that ensure easily accessible patient histories and current test results, and the availability of evidence based practice policies, procedures, and medication information resources that are essential to provide guidance for practice. Moreover there are effective systems in place which allow errors and concerns about medication processes to be reported and reviewed to improve practice [25].

Standardisation of terms, abbreviations and protocols

Many countries have recommended terminology, abbreviations and symbols that are universally accepted as good practice in the prescribing, dispensing and administration of medications [9, 11]. However, at an organisational level too it is important that there are policies and protocols documenting what is acceptable in terms of abbreviations and symbols, and then systems and processes in place to monitor compliance with these.

Other protocols that can be adopted by organisations to minimise the likelihood of error involve the adoption of 'Tall Man Letters' for drugs that look alike [14, 26]. This involves using mixed case letters to draw attention to the drug name. Examples of this are chlorproMAZINE and chlorproPAMIDE and NIFEdipine and niCARdipine. There is evidence in the literature that the highlighting of the drug names in this way captures clinicians' attention and makes it less likely there will be mix-ups [14, 26, 27]. A comprehensive list of some common drugs with similar names is available at www.ismp.org/tools/tallmanletters.pdf.

Computerised decision and medication support systems

There is a growing body of evidence that implementation of computerised medication support systems is having some impact on the incidence of errors [16, 28]. These types of systems include disease or drug specific guidelines which aid in selecting appropriate drugs, avoiding contraindicated drugs and identifying drug regime monitoring protocols [29]; computer based order entry by doctors [16]; and barcoding to enable matching of the patient's medication order with the patient and their medical information [12]. Implementing these types of systems can be met with some resistance, but there are elements that are associated with successful implementation and a reduction in errors. These include:

- ensuring computers are available at the time and location of decision making
- making it difficult to override hazard alerts
- requiring clinicians to document reasons for not following recommendations
- providing a clear display of alerts
- linking to other patient clinical data [29].

The use of a personally controlled electronic health record may also help to eliminate some errors and is probably an inevitable development in healthcare in the not too distant future. In Australia the National e-Health Transition Authority has been established to develop this process, with similar initiatives occurring in the National Health Service (NHS) in the UK, and Canada [9].

It is important to note that the introduction of any changes in processes or procedures can have unintended consequences, and can lead to different errors. In the case of computerised systems, many problems have been described involving human–machine interface flaws that have led to errors. Thus detailed ongoing analysis, modelling and usability inspections need to be in place with the introduction of these systems [20].

Storage and packaging of medications

There are several elements to this particular strategy. The first involves unit dosing so that the medications are prepared for individual patients; this has been found to reduce medication errors [8]. The second involves ensuring that medications that look alike or sound alike are not stored close to each other. The third involves removing certain medications from clinical environments. Wachter [8] cites an example of intravenous potassium, which nurses were often required to add to an IV infusion. In most instances potassium now comes in pre-mixed IV infusions.

Medication reviews by clinical pharmacists

In the hospital setting the inclusion of clinical pharmacists as part of the team looking after the patient in the clinical area has reduced errors

[8, 16]. Although pharmacists are involved in the dispensing of medication, it is relatively new to have them involved in attending patient review rounds and reviewing medication regimes at the bedside. Their presence when medications are being ordered and administered means their knowledge and expertise is immediately available to provide advice and identify potentially inappropriate medication dosages or interactions with other medication.

Patient involvement

In Chapter 2 we discussed the role that patients can and should have in their care. Patients and their families who understand their medication regime, including the dosage, the action and the side effects, can be powerful partners with clinicians in preventing medication errors. However, to include patients in the shared decision making about their care and to empower them to speak up can be challenging for both patients and clinicians.

Education

In addition to those strategies mentioned above, a vital link in the prevention of medication errors is educating all staff involved in the medication process. Understanding the organisational system factors that may increase the likelihood of errors is important. However, equally important is educating clinicians about the human factors that lead to humans making errors. Equipped with this knowledge, individuals are able to develop what Reason calls 'error wisdom' [21]. This then gives them an awareness to monitor their own practice in situations where errors are more likely to occur (see Chapter 8 for more information about the error wisdom process).

Exercise 4.3

Aim of the exercise: To match medication error prevention strategies to the different stages in the medication process.

What to do:

1. Complete the chart below, matching the error prevention strategies to the different stages in the medication process.

	Prescribing	Dispensing	Administration
Positive organisational culture			
Standardisation of terms			
Computerised decision and medication systems			
Storage and packaging of medications			
Involvement of clinical pharmacists			
Addressing short staffing			
Increasing supervision			
Wearing no-interruption vests			
Protocols for the 'five rights' of medication			
Patient involvement			
Education			

2. Can you identify other strategies from information in the sections above? If so, enter them onto this chart matching them to the different stages in the process.
3. Identify if there are particular strategies that you are able to apply or implement in your work area.
4. Discuss your findings with colleagues/friends.
5. Compare your findings with the Exercise Feedback section at the end of the chapter.

Summary

In this chapter we have reviewed the types of medication errors, the factors that lead to them and some strategies that can be utilised to reduce their likelihood. We have particularly emphasised that medication errors occur as a result of both organisational/system factors and human factors. Successful strategies to reduce medication errors need to target both areas.

The themes of this chapter relate to the WHO curriculum guideline topics of [31]:

- Why human factors are important for patient safety
- Improving medication safety.

The Exercise Feedback below provides an overview of the key points of this chapter.

EXERCISE FEEDBACK

Exercise 4.1

One notable study found that doctors do not have worse handwriting than the rest of the population [30]; nevertheless, the hazards of a poorly written prescription can have serious consequences. The contributing factors, based on our knowledge of human factor principles, include:

- busyness and the amount of writing that is required leads to illegibility and use of abbreviations
- a belief that it is essential to use symbols and acronyms to communicate with other professionals
- a lack of knowledge of the policy and procedural requirements
- a lack of awareness that handwriting is difficult to read
- as the error consequence is often remote from the prescriber, there can be a lack of feedback information about the problem being caused by the use of abbreviations and poor handwriting – diffusion of responsibility
- a culture that tolerates deviances from best practice
- a culture where other health professionals do not feel safe or empowered to challenge poor practice.

Exercise 4.2

In this situation it is important that the focus is not on blaming and shaming the student who made the error but on searching for the latent factors that led to the student giving the wrong medication. If you think back to Reason's Swiss Cheese model, the barriers that should have stopped the error were policies and protocols that detail that medication is prepared for one patient at a time and administered straightaway and include strategies to complete the 'five rights' as part of the process.

Other barriers would be ensuring that student supervisors are allocated only the number of students they can supervise directly, a strong culture that actively discourages 'workarounds' to cope with workload, and a work environment where staff do not tolerate deviations from policy and students feel safe to challenge poor practice.

Thus the factors that contributed to this incident were:

- time and efficiency pressures on supervisor that led to workaround
- culture that tolerated workarounds and deviations from policy and procedure
- authority of supervisor that put students in a situation where it was difficult to challenge poor behaviour.

Strategies that may have prevented errors include:

- lower supervisor to student ratio
- a culture that
  o understands that the checks, policies and procedures which may seem less efficient when there are time pressures actually provide the barriers to prevent human error
  o emphasises the importance of checking and the 'five rights' of medication administration
  o values best practice even when they are less efficient, and
  o where staff and students feel safe and empowered to challenge poor practice.

Exercise 4.3

Matching the error prevention strategies to the different stages in the medication process:

	Prescribing	Dispensing	Administration
Positive organisational culture	X	X	X
Standardisation of terms	X	X	X
Computerised decision and medication systems	X	X	X
Storage and packaging of medications	X	X	X
Involvement of clinical pharmacists	X	X	X
Addressing short staffing	X	X	X
Increasing supervision	X	X	X
Wearing no-interruption vests	X	X	X
Protocols for the 'five rights' of medication	X	X	X
Patient involvement	X	X	X
Education	X	X	X

You will note that the strategies identified can be applied to all stages of the medication process to prevent errors. Other strategies not listed in the table include:

- learning and practising drug calculations
- ensuring accurate medication history is obtained
- using resources to look up medications and check dosages, interactions, side effects and contraindications
- promoting good communication within the team
- reporting and learning from errors.

References

1. Schuster, P. and L. Nykolyn, *Communication for Nurses*, 2010, Philadelphia: F.A. Davis.
2. Habraken, M. and T. van der Schaff, *If only ...: Failed, missed and absent error recovery opportunities in medication errors.* Quality and Safety in Health Care, 2008. **19**(1): 37–41.
3. Yamey, G., *Family compensated for death after illegible prescription.* BMJ, 1999. **319**(7223): 1456.
4. Etchells, E., D. Juurlink, and W. Levinson, *Medication errors: The human factor.* Canadian Medical Association Journal, 2008. **178**(1).
5. Chang, Y. and B.A. Mark, *Antecedents of severe and nonsevere medication errors.* Journal of Nursing Scholarship, 2009. **41**(1): 70–78.
6. Agyemang, R.E.O. and A. While, *Medication errors: Types, causes and impact on nursing practice.* British Journal of Nursing (BJN), 2010. **19**(6): 380–385.
7. Milligan, F., *Diabetes medication incidents in the care home setting.* Nursing Standard, 2012. **26**(29): 38–43.
8. Wachter, R., *Understanding Patient Safety.* 2nd ed. 2012, San Francisco: McGraw-Hill.
9. *Recommendations for Terminology, Abbreviations and Symbols used in the Prescribing and Administration of Medicines*, 2010, Australian Commission on Safety and Quality in Healthcare.
10. *Building a Safer NHS for Patients: Improving medication safety*, 2004, Department of Health/NHS.
11. Johnson, D. and F. Johnson, *Joining Together.* 10th ed. 2010, New Jersey: Pearson.
12. Kiekkas, P., et al., *Medication errors in critically ill adults: A review of direct observation evidence.* American Journal of Critical Care, 2011. **20**(1): 36–44.
13. *Pharmacist, GP blamed for coma,* in *The Guardian*, 1988. London.
14. *FDA and IAMP lists of look-alike drug names with recommended Tall Man Letters*, 2011, ISMP.
15. Wheeler, J., et al., *The effect of drug concentration expression on epinephrine dosing errors.* Annals of Internal Medicine, 2008. **148**: 11–14.

16. Anthony, K., et al., *No interruptions please: Impact of a no interruption zone on medication safety in intensive care units [corrected] [published errata appear in CRIT CARE NURSE 2010 Aug;30(4):16, and Dec;30(6):16].* Critical Care Nurse, 2010. **30**(3): 21–30.

17. Hewitt, P., *Nurses' perceptions of the causes of medication errors: An integrative literature review.* MEDSURG Nursing, 2010. **19**(3): 159–167.

18. *ISMP Medication Safety Alert! RG Inattentional blindness: What captures your attention? ... Reprinted with permission from ISMP Medication Safety Alert! Nurse Advise-ERR (ISSN 1550-6304) August 2009 Volume 7 Issue 8 Copyright 2009 Institute for Safe Medication Practices (ISMP).* Alberta RN, 2009. **65**(8): 16–17.

19. *ISMP Medication Safety Alert! RG Shakespeare was on target – Don't be a borrower or lender ... Reprinted with permission from ISMP Medication Safety Alert! Nurse Advise-ERR (ISSN 1550-6304) May 2010 Volume 8 Issue 5 Copyright 2010 Institute for Safe Medication Practices.* Alberta RN, 2010. **66**(4): 32–34.

20. Carayon, P., ed. *Handbook of Human Factors and Ergonomics in Health Care and Patient Safety.* 2nd ed. *Human Factors and Ergonomics,* ed. G. Salvendy, 2012, Boca Raton, Florida: CRC Press.

21. Reason, J., *The Human Contribution: Unsafe acts, accidents and heroic recoveries,* 2008, Farnham, Surrey: Ashgate Publishing.

22. Ramachandran, V., *The Tell-tale Brain,* 2011, New York: Norton & Company.

23. *ISMP Medication Safety Alert! RG Patient safety should NOT be a priority in health care! ... reducing at-risk behaviours ... Reprinted with permission from ISMP Medication Safety Alert! Nurse-Advise-ERR (ISSN 1550-6304) September 2008 Volume 6 Issue 9 Copyright 2008 Institute for Safe Medication Practices.* Alberta RN, 2009. **65**(1): 23–25.

24. Reid-Searl, K., L. Moxham, and B. Happell, *Enhancing patient safety: The importance of direct supervision for avoiding medication errors and near misses by undergraduate nursing students.* International Journal of Nursing Practice, 2010. **16**(3): 225–232.

25. Choo, J., A. Hutchinson, and T. Bucknall, *Nurses' role in medication safety.* Journal of Nursing Management, 2010. **18**(7): 853–861.

26. Filik, R., et al., *Labeling of medicines and patient safety: Evaluating methods of reducing drug name confusion.* Human Factors, 2006. **48**(1): 39–47.

27. Robertson, A., et al., *Implementation and adoption of nationwide electronic health records in secondary care in England: Qualitative analysis of interim results from a prospective national evaluation.* BMJ, 2010. **341**: 871–893.

28. Howard, R. and A. Avery, *Medicines management,* in *Health Care Errors and Patient Safety,* B. Hurwitz and A. Sheikh, eds. 2009, Oxford: Wiley-Blackwell.

29. Avery, A., A. Sheikh, and B. Hurwitz, *Safer medicines management in primary care.* British Journal of General Practice, 2002. **52**: S17–S22.

30. Schneider, K., C. Murray, R. Shadduck, and D. Meyers, *Legibility of doctors' handwriting is as good (or bad) as everyone else's.* Quality and Safety in Health Care, 2006. **15**(6): 445.

31. *WHO Patient Safety Curriculum Guide: Multi-professional edition,* 2011, Geneva: World Health Organization.

5

Teamwork and Patient Safety

Introduction

A team is described as 'a group of people who work together towards a shared and meaningful outcome in ways that combine their individual skills and abilities and for which they are all responsible' [1]. The importance of healthcare teams functioning effectively is growing with the effects of increasing complexity of care required, along with the rise of co-morbidities and chronic disease, resulting in the involvement of many people in the provision of care for any one person. The impact of workforce shortages and introduction of safe working hours initiatives also highlights the need for effective teamwork [2]. The number of people who can potentially be involved in the care of a patient for one episode of care could include several teams of doctors (primary healthcare general practice, general medical physicians, general surgeons and all of the different specialty medical and surgical specialties); many different general nurses as well as specialty nurses, community nurses and mental health nurses; allied health including physiotherapists, dietitians and social workers; and possibly various other groups too numerous to mention here. It is clear that unless this group of people cooperate with one another, communicate effectively and coordinate the care process, the potential for errors is enormous.

In this chapter we will first look at the importance of effective teamwork for safety and quality outcomes for patients. We will then discuss the attributes of an effective team and the barriers to achieving this. We will look at some strategies and tools that can be adopted by organisations and individuals to improve teamwork, and examine in more detail key areas for effective team communication including structured communication tools, and protocols for the handover of care.

Teamwork and Patient Safety

There is considerable research supporting the view that teamwork, and specifically coordination and communication within the team, plays an integral part in maintaining patient safety [3–9]. In Western Australia it was identified in the 2005/06 Sentinel Event report that 25 per cent of sentinel events involved poor communication. The results were similar for 2006/07 [10, 11]. The Accident and Incident (AIMS) data for Western Australia 2001–2007 report identified that communication issues were a significant factor in 21 per cent of critical incidents [12]. This type of data is not specific to one country but is similar across different health systems. In the US a Joint Commission Study of over 3000 events indicated that communication failures were the identified cause for 665 of them [13].

In a study examining teamwork and errors during a neonatal resuscitation, the researchers studied the resuscitation events using a video recording [14]. Teamwork behaviours such as information sharing, inquiry, sharing intentions, evaluating plans, managing workload and teaching/advising were coded for each event. The researchers found that where these behaviours were prevalent within the team there were fewer errors. Other clinical studies in the operating room [15], emergency departments [16] and trauma resuscitation [17] have all found that poor teamwork is associated with compromised quality of patient care. Effective teamwork is not only essential in the acute care hospital setting but also essential for optimal patient outcomes in other settings such as community care, the aged care sector, primary care and mental health [18]. Consider an emergency scenario where the team leader is barking instructions to the rest of the team, assigning roles and then immediately reassigning them to others, asking several people to do the same task and constantly asking for information from people without listening to their responses. It is not hard to appreciate that this team would not be functioning effectively.

The understanding that the care of patients can span many teams leads us to appreciate that effective teamwork is not limited to a single team but is also crucial in the communication and handovers between teams. Examples of this are when one shift of clinicians transfers responsibility for care to the next shift, or when a patient is moved between acute care and chronic care, or hospital care and community care. In one study 12 per cent of patients experienced an adverse event after discharge mainly related to poor communication about medication regimes [19]. Another study identified that nearly 50 per cent of patients have examination results such as blood tests or X-rays waiting to be reported when they are discharged. This leads to the situation where many of the results are not communicated to the patient's community care team and thus they are not actioned appropriately [20].

When a healthcare team is not working effectively as a team, patient safety is compromised because there is the potential for poor coordination of care, failed communication related to the patient's condition and treatment orders, and for information to be misinterpreted [21]. In the next section we will look at the attributes that make up an effective team.

Effective Teamwork Characteristics

Individuals make up a team. A well-functioning individual team member is constantly recognising cues in the environment, acquiring contextual information from other sources, remembering information and processing all of this to plan and execute actions [22]. To function as a team the individuals within the team must utilise the information they gather to act in a collective fashion. This is called shared cognition [10] and enables effective teams to coordinate, cooperate and communicate to make decisions, plan and undertake the tasks required of them.

Coordination involves the team working together to plan and manage the actions that are required to complete the task(s). The actions need to be orchestrated, synchronised and combined if clinicians' contributions, time and resources are to be used efficiently and effectively and for optimal outcomes for patients [10].

Cooperation is the second requirement for teams to function effectively. Team members must have the motivation and desire to work together. Cooperation requires all team members to have a shared understanding of the roles and responsibilities. This leads to trust and respect for the capabilities, contribution and performance of other team members [10, 23].

Effective communication is the third element of good teamwork and relies on the exchange of information between the sender and the receiver. It should be noted that communication is not just the words that are used in verbal communication – body language, tone and attitude can also influence the message received. Communication also involves the exchange of written information [23].

When communication within the healthcare team is not effective, there is a risk of compromised patient safety. Team members are not passive but actively process information and they do this through their own filters and understanding. Knowing that people are active recipients of the messages from others means we must check they have received the message that was intended. Shared understanding underpins the process of cooperation. The importance of good communication in teams to facilitate coordination and cooperation is paramount.

Effective teams do not just happen – each of the elements of coordination, cooperation and communication require specific behaviours from team members. The behaviours are summarised in Table 5.1.

Table 5.1 Effective teamwork behaviours that support the key functions of a team

Team action	Required behaviours
Coordination	Team members: • have a common purpose • have a common understanding of the task and the resources available • have a clear understanding of all team member roles and responsibilities • observe and correct where required other team members' actions • provide and request assistance when required • recognise other team members' good performance • compensate for other team members when required • review team effectiveness and adjust actions as required • provide feedback to each other • distribute and assign tasks according to requirements of the task.
Cooperation	Team members: • put team goals ahead of personal goals • resolve conflict effectively • have confidence and trust in other team members' intentions • can adjust to, adapt and anticipate actions of other team members • back up each other to complete actions and tasks.
Communication	Team members: • seek information from all resources • share information with the rest of the team and individual team members as required in a timely manner • communicate using accepted procedures and proper terminology, concisely and audibly • acknowledge communication and check for correct interpretation.

Adapted from Wilson (2007) and Miller (2010) [24, 25].

Baker et al. [10] identify several skills, knowledge areas and attributes that combine into the individual competencies which contribute to an effective team. These include:

- leadership – the competency to direct, plan, organise and coordinate activities (TL)
- situation monitoring – the competency to achieve a common understanding of the situation and task at hand in order to be able to monitor team effectiveness and required actions (S)
- mutual support – the competencies to be able to understand and anticipate other team members' needs (MS)
- adaptability – the competency to be able to recognise and action the need to shift resources as required to respond to changing conditions (A)
- shared mental models – the competency to understand the requirements of the task in relation to how team members interact (SMM)
- communication – the competency to utilise the components of effective communication appropriately (C)
- collective orientation – the competency to identify and give priority to the contribution of others to the whole team and team goals (CO)
- mutual trust – the reciprocated belief that others in the team will act in the interest of the team goals (MT) [10].

Exercise 5.1

Aim of the exercise: To assess your individual competencies in relation to your contribution as a member of a team, past or present.

What to do:

1. Each of the following statements describes a behaviour that demonstrates a competency that contributes to effective teamwork. Choose a team that you are currently a member of or have been in the past (it doesn't have to be a healthcare team). Think about how you function within that team and then rate how you think you function (or have functioned) in your chosen team using the following scale:

    5 = I always behave that way
    4 = I frequently behave that way
    3 = I occasionally behave that way
    2 = I seldom behave that way
    1 = I never behave that way

A. I facilitate team problem solving (TL) _____
B. I identify the opportunities for improvement and innovation (A) _____
C. I recognise when there is a workload distribution problem within the team (MS) _____
D. I identify slips, lapses and mistakes in other team members' actions (S) _____
E. I identify changes in the team or task, and adjust strategies as needed (SMM) _____
F. I follow up with team members to ensure the message has been received (C) _____
G. I am willing to admit mistakes and accept feedback (MT) _____
H. I seek and evaluate information that impacts on team functioning (TL) _____
I. I engage in team feedback meetings (TL) _____
J. I clarify that the message I have received is the same as the intended message sent (C) _____
K. I listen to and evaluate alternative solutions proposed by other team members to plan team actions or solve task/situation problems (CO) _____
L. I remain vigilant to changes in the context, environment or situation, and develop new plans to manage the changes (MS) _____

Adapted from Baker et al. (2006) and Johnson and Johnson (2010) [10, 26].

2. Note the letters in brackets after each statement. These refer to a particular competency identified in the section above. Now review your scores for each of the competencies. Areas of competency that require development for you are those that have a lower score of the possible total for that particular competency.
3. Repeat this exercise thinking about a different team you have been a member of and compare the scores for each of the competencies in these different teams. Note any similarities and differences in how you function in the teams. What if anything do these scores suggest to you about your team functioning? Are there things you would like to do in a different way in the future?
4. Add up your total score for all competencies for both tests and then compare them with colleagues who have completed this

exercise. Note any similarities and differences in how you function in teams.

5. Discuss your results with friends and colleagues. Were there any surprises? Can you identify factors that could account for the similarities and differences in the different teams? What have you learnt about your own style of contributing to teamwork that will be useful to take into your own work?

6. Compare your findings with the Exercise Feedback section at the end of the chapter.

A fundamental feature of a successful team is effective leadership. The role of the leader is to bring the team together by providing coordination of the team activities and facilitating cooperation and communication. This involves having an overview of the dynamic situation, setting priorities, decision making, using the resources both efficiently and effectively, and encouraging and mentoring the team [27]. In a healthcare setting the leader may be a designated leader (e.g. physician in charge, the nurse leader, the surgeon in theatre). However, the leader may be an assumed leader who takes on the role given their knowledge or particular skills that meet the requirements for the situation in question [28–30]. Effective team leaders need to be able to:

- balance authority and assertiveness with encouraging team members' participation
- plan and coordinate required tasks
- utilise available resources efficiently
- delegate to other team members
- manage and resolve conflict
- manage errors in a constructive way to maintain team functioning [31].

While team leaders are a vital component of successful teams, every member of the team is required to contribute if the team is to achieve optimum performance.

Having identified the competencies and behaviours that support effective teamwork, we will now move on to examine barriers to the development of effective teams.

Barriers to Effective Teamwork

We have noted previously that there are many health professionals involved in any one patient's care. However, because of the nature of health professionals' work, most health professionals tend to work autonomously to carry out their particular part of the patient's care. That said, even though they work autonomously, their part of the patient care cannot stand alone, but forms part of the whole package of patient care. On the whole, most clinicians recognise this, and the need to work together as a team, but there are pervasive barriers that contribute to misunderstandings and difficulties in communication, coordination and cooperation [32, 33]. Some of these problems are general barriers that can occur in any context and therefore are not particular to healthcare. Other barriers are directly related to the way healthcare is organised and structured. A sound understanding of the barriers is a prerequisite for recognising, acknowledging and addressing them.

The general barriers to effective teamwork can relate to differences in gender, language, generation, culture, ethnicity and personality types [23]. Any of these can result in misunderstandings and incorrect perceptions of meaning related to communication between different individuals who do not share a common background. Generational difficulties can impact on the formation and maintenance of effective teams because of different communication styles, perceptions of respect for position and age, changes in technology and also differing expectations of work experience and responsibilities [34].

These general barriers affect teams in the healthcare context and can serve as impediments to effective teamwork. There are also specific features of the healthcare context that can result in poor teamwork. In the main these are associated with the way the different health professionals relate to each other and the sometimes opposing expectations of what the primary goal is in patient care.

A healthcare professional's scope and focus of practice result in having different perceptions of the care provided and what patients may require. Some of these perceptions arise from a different focus of their education. For example, with the medical profession the focus of the patient care is the treatment, whether that be cure or to 'fix the problem'. Treatments are based on science and evidence, and communication with colleagues about patients is concise and informed by the facts. On the other hand, nurses' education emphasises the caring needs of the patient linked to treatment. To provide this caring requires an extensive education based also on science and evidence that underpins the nursing decisions about patient care. This different emphasis in the main leads to a communication style that is different to doctors, being of a broader, more narrative style [9]. Thus when doctors and nurses communicate, misunderstandings can arise because the doctor can feel the nurse is not getting to the point and the nurse feels the doctor is being impatient and rushing the communication.

There is no definitive evidence on the prevalence of failure to communicate in teams as a factor in healthcare errors, but in other industries such as aviation failure to communicate was the most common type of communication failure [31]. Given the similarities in barriers to effective communication such as steep authority gradients arising from the hierarchical nature of healthcare teams (see below) and the fragmented nature of healthcare planning identified in previous chapters, it is very likely that failure to communicate is a major factor in errors in healthcare. These *failure to communicate* situations can arise because of a deliberate decision not to communicate, not realising that communication was required or because of distractions or absentmindedness [31]. Communication failures may also occur because there is a lack of information, incorrect information, too much information or non-verbal cues are inappropriate causing the message content to be misunderstood [23, 31, 35].

Let us examine in some more detail the potential communication failures linked to the hierarchical system in healthcare. As noted previously, healthcare is a very hierarchical system, with doctors generally being seen as the top and other team members as being further down the hierarchy. This results in what is known as an authority gradient, where those who perceive themselves – or are perceived by others – as being lower down the hierarchy feel powerless to challenge or ask questions of those who are more senior. Hierarchical lines of communication with steep authority gradients can involve waiting for orders, unquestioning compliance with directives, and disincentives to questioning and raising concerns. Conversely, where teams demonstrate a low authority gradient, staff are more likely to raise concerns and discuss observations – thus errors are more likely to be prevented and patient safety improved [9].

An example of this is an actual situation where a four-year-old boy received facial burns during maxillofacial surgery as a result of a dry swab placed on his face by the maxillofacial surgeon catching fire during the application of diathermy. The maxillofacial surgeon had not realised this was a risk and immediately changed his practice, using moistened swabs instead. He subsequently learnt that the theatre nurses were aware of the risks, as the other maxillofacial surgeons routinely used moist swabs in this type of surgery. When he asked why they had not raised the issue with him they explained that when they had tried to raise issues like this in the past with surgeons they had been rebuffed in such a manner that they were now very reluctant to make any suggestions to change surgical practice [31].

Another situation that can lead to communication failure is when the person receiving the message does not realise there is a time critical or non-routine element to the message. This can occur in emergency situations or when there is a change of plan (such as change in the scheduling of theatre cases in the operating room). To illustrate this situation, one study in Bristol asked a range of doctors at differing levels of seniority to identify the urgency of pages they received. The way they rated urgency was to ignore the message until they got a second page from the same ward which they perceived might indicate the message was urgent [36].

Communication failures can also occur when the sender of the message fails to appreciate that the person receiving the message may be distracted. This can occur because the receiver is engaged in a focused, time critical or emergency activity, or when there is a lot of environmental distraction (e.g. noise). Of particular importance in healthcare is to appreciate that this can also happen when the receiver is fatigued or woken from a deep sleep [31, 37].

Strategies to Improve Teamwork

In Chapter 4 we looked at organisational/structural strategies that could be implemented to decrease the likelihood of medication errors. In particular we discussed the impact of a positive organisational culture, standardisation of terms and protocols, human resource management and education. These broad organisational strategies are also factors in supporting the development of effective teamwork. Most importantly, and a crucial first step, is for organisations to recognise the importance of teamwork to effective and safe patient outcomes.

Moreover, acknowledging the impact of the hierarchical nature of relationships in healthcare and the negative consequences this has on teamwork is vital if organisational leaders are going to establish and model the behaviours to break down the communication problems which can result from it. Policies and protocols backed up by systems that deal with inappropriate communication behaviour indicate to all staff that questioning and challenging treatment plans and decisions is acceptable and encouraged to promote safety within the organisation. Acknowledging and including the patient and their family as a member of the team is another important strategy for improving teamwork and thus patient safety. Providing information about their healthcare and medication plans to patients means that if necessary they can ensure other health professionals involved in their care are informed of them. As noted in Chapter 2, providing the opportunity for patients to read their own medical records gives them the chance to correct any mistaken information.

Education and training in teamwork behaviours has been shown to improve team effectiveness [13, 34, 38]. There are different types of training foci. These include cross-training, where team members are trained on other team members' roles and responsibilities; procedural training, where the team is trained to follow a standard sequence of actions to be followed in a given set of circumstances; and perturbation training, which focuses on presenting teams with different and varying situations which requires team skills in coordination, collaboration and communication as they manage each one [21].

Another training programme which has been shown to be particularly effective in the healthcare environment has been adapted from the crew resource management (CRM) aviation programmes [23]. Aviation has been shown to have particular similarities to healthcare in terms of the hierarchical structure of teams and the interprofessional relationships [9]. The CRM programme focuses on trust, respect, communication, appropriate assertiveness and shared decision making and so is particularly useful for breaking down the barriers and building effective teamwork in healthcare, with some studies showing a 20 per cent improvement in team performance after undergoing CRM training [38].

The introduction of structured communication protocols and policies and standardised tools have also been shown to improve the accuracy and understanding of the information being shared between professionals and the effectiveness of teamwork [23]. The communication tools can be used as a prompt in different scenarios. Although the tools work optimally when they are adopted by organisations, and everyone within those organisations is trained and understands them, they can still be used by individuals without organisational support as a means to structure their communication.

These tools provide a structured approach to ensure that the content of any message delivered is organised in a logical way that lessens the likelihood of misunderstandings. They focus on using objective, concise information about the patient and thus offer a mechanism to use appropriate assertion in challenging situations without the emotion that can arise from a lack of a shared mental model or hierarchical structures that can block effective communication [9, 23, 32, 39]. Three communication processes – SBAR (Situation, Background, Assessment, Recommendation), CUS (Concerned, Uncomfortable, Safety Issue), and structured handover protocols – are reviewed briefly in the following sections.

SBAR (Situation, Background, Assessment, Recommendation)

The SBAR tool was developed to provide a framework for clinicians to communicate their concerns about a patient. It is simple to use and has been shown with practice to be highly effective in increasing the quality of communication between team members [39].

SBAR structures the communication as follows:

- **Situation:** What is going on with the patient?
- **Background:** What is the clinical background or context?
- **Assessment:** What do I think the problem is?
- **Recommendation/Response:** What do I think needs to be done to correct the problem in what timeframe?

For example:
Good morning Dr X, I am a nurse on 9th floor. I am ringing about your patient Mr Jones. He is reporting increasing abdominal pain of 8 out of 10 unrelieved by pain relief delivered by PCA (patient controlled analgesia). This pain is associated with increasing restlessness, diaphoresis (profuse sweating), tachycardia of 140 bpm, hypotension of 70/40, and poor urine output in the last few hours of less than 20 mls an hour. There is minimal drainage from his wound, but his abdomen is tense and swollen. He has IV saline 9% infusing at 50 mls an hour **(Situation)**. Mr Jones is the 50-year-old man who had open prostatectomy surgery yesterday who has no other significant past medical history **(Background)**. I am concerned that he may be bleeding internally **(Assessment)**. I would like to increase his IV fluid regime and would appreciate it if you could review him in the next 5 minutes **(Recommendation)**.

Structuring your communication this way takes practice and certainly requires the use of critical thinking skills. Studies have identified that there is some hesitancy initially, on the part of a nurse, to provide the 'recommendation' to doctors but this is overcome with time and familiarity with the process [39]. Remember your recommendation may ultimately prove to be incorrect, but stating this as part of SBAR communication provides the person you are talking to with your definition of the problem based on objective data and provides the context for your concern for a timely response.

Exercise 5.2

Aim of the exercise: To provide you with the opportunity to practise SBAR communication. Ideally this exercise should be completed with two or more people, but if this is not possible then complete the exercise on your own but find the opportunity to discuss and compare your results with others.

What to do:

1. Read the following case study and then answer the questions.

   A 55-year-old obese woman with a history of hypertension and severe obstructive sleep apnea requiring CPAP (continuous positive airway pressure) is placed on morphine PCA (patient-controlled anaesthesia) pump for pain control following cholecystectomy. At approximately 1:00 AM, 5 hours after starting the morphine, the patient's respiratory rate decreased to 7 (while on CPAP). Physical examination revealed an oxygen saturation level of 98%, normal blood pressure, heart rate of 50, and pinpoint pupils. The patient was noted to be lethargic, opening her eyes and mumbling incoherently in response to vigorous shaking but quickly falling asleep when the stimulus ceased. Concerned, the RN called the attending physician and stated that 'the patient was sleepy and difficult to rouse'. The physician seemed annoyed by the call, barking, 'What would you expect when you wake up a patient in the middle of the night from deep sleep – an excellent level of consciousness? Naturally, she would be drowsy!' He followed with, 'Wake me up only on life and death issues!'

   Reprinted with permission of AHRQ WebM&M. Source: Duffy D, Cassel CK. Do not disturb! AHRQ WebM&M [serial online]. October 2007. Available at: www.webmm.ahrq.gov/case.aspx?caseID=161.

2. Identify some reasons that may have caused the doctor to react this way.
3. Using the SBAR tool make notes of how you could communicate to the doctor your concern about this patient's condition.

4. Discuss and compare your SBAR communication plan with colleagues.
5. Compare your findings with the Exercise Feedback section at the end of the chapter.

You may also find that if you adopt this technique of communicating your concerns there is no encouragement from other team members, even to the point of being rebuffed. However, it is important to remember that objective communication is in the interest of patient safety, and using SBAR moves communication away from personalities to the patient issue or problem that needs addressing. It is acknowledged throughout the literature that the common custom of speaking indirectly, described by Haig [39] as the 'hint and hope' method of communication, carries the highest risk of a compromised outcome for patients [3, 8, 10, 14, 23, 25, 33, 39].

The SBAR tool is not limited to use as a verbal tool – it is also useful to frame written communications between clinicians to ensure that all information is conveyed to other team members. SBAR can also form the basis of a written or verbal handover tool; we will explore this in greater depth below. But first we will discuss the CUS communication tool.

CUS (Concerned, Uncomfortable, Safety Issue)

The CUS tool is a technique that was developed as part of the crew resource management training [40, 41]. It is a communication method that provides an objective way for someone lower in the hierarchy to get the attention of someone higher up, in serious safety situations. CUS is a three stage escalating process for getting attention when you have safety concerns. It involves the following prompts:

- I am **concerned** ...
- I am **uncomfortable** ...
- This is a **safety issue** ... .

The use of this tool is not limited to the acute hospital setting; it can be applied across multiple contexts including aged care, community care, mental health, primary care and general practice. An example of successful adoption in the community is the Berwick Home Health & Hospice Service in New York, where the Home nurses use it when they feel their concerns about a patient are not being acted upon in a timely manner [42].

Like the SBAR tool mentioned above, CUS works better when adopted as a communication strategy across an organisation. However, even if this is not the case, you as an individual practitioner or manager can use it to objectively raise concerns. The scaled escalation of your concern identifies that you do not consider the issue a trivial one, and that you are seeking action immediately. You may need to bypass the individual who is dismissing your concerns and raise the issue with someone more senior. Continue to use the structured protocols if required, as the focus will then remain on the patient's safety rather than the professional behaviour of the individuals involved. It is important though to ensure that the words have their intended impact by only using this tool in situations of time critical patient safety concerns.

Exercise 5.3

Aim of the exercise: To practise the use of the CUS tool.

What to do:

1. Using the case study in the previous exercise (5.2) make the assumption that you have used the SBAR tool to communicate with the doctor your concern about this patient. However, your concerns are still dismissed. Using the CUS tool develop a communication plan that details your escalating concerns.
2. If the CUS communication plan does not get the outcome you are looking for, what other strategies could you utilise?
3. Discuss your plans with colleagues. In your discussion identify the possible effects of introducing this type of communication into your work. How might this change your view of yourself as a professional and how others might see you?
4. Compare your findings with the Exercise Feedback section at the end of the chapter.

Handover protocols

The final area we are going to look at in this chapter on effective teamwork and communication is handover protocols. Different organisations use a range of terminology to describe the transition of patient care from one clinician or team to another, including handoff, sign-out, sign-over and shift change report. We will use the term handover and use this to describe the transferring of patient information (and responsibility and accountability) from one clinician to another to enable ongoing safe, effective and timely care of that patient.

There are two types of patient handover. The first involves the handover of care when a patient moves between different contexts, for example from the operating theatre to the ward, or from the hospital to the care of the general practitioner in the community, or from an aged care facility to an acute care hospital. The second involves the handover of information between different caregivers providing the care for the particular episode of care, for example between the day shift and night shift (in the main nursing and medical staff), or the medical team and allied health team such as physiotherapist, dietician or pharmacist, or the many different clinical specialists who may be involved in the patient's care [35].

Handover errors are the most common in healthcare [9, 35, 43, 44]. Friesen et al. [44] noted that the issues which contribute to errors in handover are a lack of structured communication policies or protocols leading to failed communication, omissions, distractions, absence of or illegible documentation and use of transfer forms, incomplete medical records, limited access to information and poor knowledge on the part of clinicians about effective handover techniques.

An effective handover requires that the clinician who is accepting responsibility and accountability for the patient care has a clear understanding of the current status of the patient. This will also include an awareness of any previous or current healthcare issues that might affect assessment and understanding of the patient's condition or potential changes in condition and requirements, and who is responsible for ongoing treatment and care [35]. Best practice recommendations include the use of a standardised tool for the handover of care, allowing time for asking and answering questions, checking understanding by repeating back key points, and limiting interruptions and distractions [45, 46]. These recommendations reinforce and support a more effective handover.

Individual clinicians can structure their written or verbal handover of care using any of the variety of tools available. Searching the internet using the terms 'patient handover guidelines/tools' will provide you with many examples. As with the communication tools discussed above, these handover tools work much better when they are adopted and supported across an organisation, However, even in the absence of this support, you as an individual can 'be the change you want to see'

(Mahatma Gandhi, 1869–1948) and provide individual leadership in ensuring effective handover that maximises the quality of care and safety for patients. The SBAR tool we discussed above in relation to communication can also be used to structure handover information as follows [43]:

- **Situation:** What is the situation? (current patient condition/ diagnosis)
- **Background:** What is the clinical background? (previous history or recent treatment)
- **Assessment:** What is the current status? (vital signs, other observations, test results, symptoms)
- **Recommendation:** What needs to be done, by whom and when? (ongoing care, tests and monitoring, discharge, escalation plan).

Another example is the 'SHARED' (Situation, History, Assessment, Risks, Expectation and Documentation) tool [43]. This tool structures the handover as follows:

- **Situation:** Current patient condition or diagnosis
- **History:** Previous history or recent treatment
- **Assessment:** Current status, vital signs, test results, symptoms
- **Risks:** Allergies, falls, pressure areas, infection control, socio-cultural
- **Expectation:** Ongoing care, tests and monitoring, discharge, escalation plan
- **Documentation:** Progress notes, care pathways, observations.

These are just two of the tools that can be used and a cursory search of the internet will elicit many others you can examine for your own clinical area.

Exercise 5.4

Aim of the exercise: To identify the different handover failures and the impact on effective teamwork.

What to do:

1. Read the following case study and then answer the questions.

   Mrs Jones, aged 75 years, was admitted to a rehabilitation ward following hip surgery for a fracture sustained in a fall at home. The transfer sheet between the acute hospital and rehabilitation hospital was not completed as there had been a verbal handover of the patient's condition between nursing staff by telephone on the morning of the transfer, but no social history was passed on.

Mrs Jones was a widow and lived alone. Although she had a supportive family they did not live close and were unable to help with daily activities.

The rehabilitation unit was a very busy unit particularly understaffed with Allied Health staff who struggled with their workloads. The physiotherapist who assessed all patients on admission habitually made notes in a notebook about each patient and then wrote them up formally at the end of her shift. In this case the physiotherapist mistakenly wrote that Mrs Jones had a partner whom she lived with who helped her with her activities.

As part of the rehabilitation programme a social worker reviewed Mrs Jones to identify if there was a need for home support. Reading the physiotherapist's note to ascertain Mrs Jones' physical capabilities she noted that Mrs Jones had a partner who was able to help her. Due to her heavy workload and her assumption that Mrs Jones did not need help as she had a partner, the social worker assumed Mrs Jones was a low priority and thus did not have the opportunity to review her before her discharge home, but she noted on the discharge summary to the local District Nursing Service that Mrs Jones did not need home support.

On discharge Mrs Jones struggled with managing the activities of daily living as she did not have anyone to help her and subsequently was readmitted to the local hospital with poor nutritional status and dehydration.

2. Identify the handover failures in this scenario.
3. Using the SBAR and SHARED handover tools, identify the information that should have been handed over about this patient.
4. Discuss your findings with colleagues. Identify how you could apply your findings to situations that you may encounter in the future.
5. Compare your findings with the Exercise Feedback section at the end of the chapter.

Other protocols that can be adopted by organisations to support effective teamwork communication include protocols for structured handovers between clinicians, different clinical departments and the different healthcare sectors such as acute care, primary care and aged care, all of whom may be involved in the ongoing care of the patient.

These protocols can take the form of written 'cue sheets' or formal documentation that has been agreed by all stakeholders involved as meeting the information needs of each [46].

Implementing any or all of these strategies to improve teamwork across an organisation can be very challenging. They all require the commitment of resources, strong organisational leadership, stakeholder engagement and an implementation and evaluation plan [23, 43, 45]. We will examine these aspects in greater detail in Chapter 8.

Summary

Our focus in this chapter has been on understanding the importance of teamwork and identifying the characteristics and competencies of effective teams. We also examined factors that influence effective teamwork and identified strategies, including specific structured communication tools, that can be utilised by organisations to improve teamwork. Effective teamwork results in fewer errors and fewer adverse events.

The themes of this chapter relate to the WHO curriculum guideline topic of [2]:

• Being an effective team player.

The Exercise Feedback below provides an overview of the key points of this chapter.

EXERCISE FEEDBACK

Exercise 5.1

Your responses to this exercise will be personal to your own experiences. There are no right or wrong answers. However, we hope this exercise has enabled you to think about where you might focus in relation to your own teamwork skills and competency development. These skills and competencies are listed again below:

• leadership
• situation monitoring
• mutual support
• adaptability

- shared mental model
- communication
- collective orientation
- mutual trust.

Exercise 5.2

There are several reasons why the physician may have reacted in this negative manner and not appreciated the importance of the communication. The general barriers to effective communication can be a result of differences between the two people communicating including:

- gender, language, generation, culture, ethnicity and personality types.

Or the issue with the communication may have been related to barriers more specific to the health context. These may have included:

- contrasting scope and focus of practice which tends to lead to differing communication styles – nursing narrative style versus medical concise and factual
- authority gradients between medical and nursing staff
- the physician being fatigued and woken from sleep not realising the importance of the message.

A more effective way to communicate the message using SBAR would be for the RN to state clearly:

> Good evening Dr. I am ringing you as I am concerned about the patient MRS … . The **situation** is that the patient's respiratory rate has decreased to 7 while on CPAP. Her blood pressure is normal, heart rate is 50, and her oxygen saturation is 98%. She has pinpoint pupils, responding to vigorous stimuli by opening her eyes and mumbling but quickly falls asleep when stimulus is ceased. The **background** is that this lady has a history of hypertension, and severe sleep apnea, and following a cholecystectomy today she is on a morphine infusion that was commenced 5 hours ago. My **assessment** is that the patient has developed respiratory depression secondary to the narcotic infusion and I would like you to assess her immediately with the view to ceasing or reducing the infusion **(recommendation)**.

Exercise 5.3

Assuming that the physician has rebuffed you after using the SBAR tool you could then utilise the CUS tool. So the conversation would continue …

*Dr, I am **concerned** about this patient's condition ... I am **uncomfortable** with your refusal to review this patient ... I believe that this is a **safety issue** and needs immediate action.*

If you were still unable to get action then you would need to escalate your concerns to more senior colleagues. Many organisations include in their protocols for the management of deteriorating patients escalation procedures detailing exactly who to contact in a situation where you have been unable to get assistance for a patient you are concerned about.

Exercise 5.4

Using the SBAR and SHARED handover tools identify the information that should have been handed over about this patient
In this situation a verbal handover without supporting documentation in the form of some transfer sheet is unacceptable. The nurse who took the handover would be relying on memory or short notes to document this adequately on the arrival of Mrs Jones to the ward. Without the cues on the transfer sheet much of the information the two nurses may not have discussed some of the important information about Mrs Jones on the telephone. This is demonstrated by the omission of the social history. Using either the SBAR or Shared format may have reduced this likelihood but does not obviate the need for the information to have been documented on a transfer sheet that arrived with the patient. The error made by the physiotherapist in documenting the social history was compounded when the Social Worker, due to her heavy workload, was unable to validate or discuss the information with Mrs Jones, thus the information on her discharge summary was incorrect and lead to a compromise in patient safety that resulted in an admission to hospital.

Using the SBAR format the following information should have been included in the handover:

- **Situation:** What is the situation? (current patient condition/ diagnosis)
- **Background:** What is the clinical background? (previous history or recent treatment)
- **Assessment:** What is the current status? (vital signs, other observations, test results, symptoms)
- **Recommendation:** What needs to be done, by whom and when? (ongoing care, tests and monitoring, discharge, escalation plan).

Using the SHARED format the following information should been included in the handover:

- **Situation:** Current patient condition or diagnosis
- **History:** Previous history or recent treatment
- **Assessment:** Current status, vital signs, test results, symptoms
- **Risks:** Allergies, falls, pressure areas, infection control, socio-cultural
- **Expectation:** Ongoing care, tests and monitoring, discharge, and escalation plan
- **Documentation:** progress notes, care pathways, observations.

References

1. Baguley, P., *Teams and Team-working*, 2002, London: Hodder and Stoughton.
2. *WHO Patient Safety Curriculum Guide: Multi-professional edition*, 2011, Geneva: World Health Organization.
3. IOM, *Keeping Patients Safe: Transforming the work environment of nurses*, 2004, Washington, DC: National Academy Press.
4. Kirk, S., et al., *Evaluating safety culture*, in *Patient Safety: Research into practice*, K. Walshe and R. Boaden, eds. 2006, Maidenhead, Berkshire: Open University Press: 173–184.
5. Leape, L., *Patient safety: What have we learned? Where are we going?* in *4th Australasian Conference on Safety and Quality in Health Care*. 2006, Melbourne, Australia.
6. McClure, M. and A. Hinshaw, eds. *Magnet Hospitals Revisited*. 3rd ed. 2002, Washington: American Nurses Publishing.
7. McLean, J. and M. Walsh, *Lessons from the Inquiry into Obstetrics and Gynaecology Services at King Edward Memorial Hospital 1990–2000*. Australian Health Review, 2003. **26**: 12–23.
8. Miller, L.A., *Patient safety and teamwork in perinatal care*. Journal of Perinatal and Neonatal Nursing, 2005. **19**(1): 46–51.
9. Wachter, R., *Understanding Patient Safety*, 2012, San Francisco: McGraw-Hill.
10. Baker, P., R. Day, and E. Salas, *Teamwork as an essential component of high-reliability organizations. (Public Policy and Research Agenda)*. Health Services Research, 2006. **41**(4): 1576–1598.
11. *Delivering Safety Health Care in WA: WA Sentinel Event Report 2006–2007* [accessed 23 February 2009]. Available from: www.health.gov.au.
12. Gillespie, B.M., W. Chaboyer, and A. Lizzio, *Teamwork in the OR: Enhancing communication through team-building interventions*. ACORN, 2008. **21**(1): 14, 16, 18–19.
13. O'Leary, K., et al., *Patterns of nurse–physician communication and agreement on the plan of care*. Quality and Safety in Health Care, 2010. **19**: 195–199.

14. Williams, A., R. Lasky, and J. Dannemiller, *Teamwork behaviours and errors during neonatal resuscitation.* Quality and Safety in Health Care, 2010. **19**: 60–64.

15. Makary, M., J. Sexton, and J. Freischlag, *Operating room teamwork among physicians and nurses: Teamwork in the eye of the beholder.* Journal of the American College of Surgeons, 2006. **202**: 746–752.

16. Morey, J., R. Simon, and G. Jay, *Error reduction and performance improvement in the emergency department through formal teamwork training: Evaluation results of the medteam project.* Health Services Management Research, 2002. **37**: 1553–1581.

17. Santora, T., S. Trooskin, and C. Blank, *Video assessment of trauma response: Adherence to ATLS protocols.* American Journal of Emergency Medicine, 1996. **14**: 564–569.

18. Pearce, S., F. Watts, and A. Watkins, *Team performance, communication and patient safety,* in *Patient Safety: Research into practice,* K. Walshe and R. Boaden, eds. 2006, Maidenhead, Berkshire: Open University Press.

19. Forster, A., H. Murff, and J. Peterson, *The incidence and severity of adverse events affecting patients after discharge from hospital.* Annals of Internal Medicine, 2003. **138**: 161–167.

20. Roy, C., E. Poon, and A. Karson, *Patient safety concerns arising from test results that return after hospital discharge.* Annals of Internal Medicine, 2005. **143**: 121–128.

21. Gorman, J.C., N.J. Cooke, and P.G. Amazeen, *Training adaptive teams.* Human Factors: The Journal of the Human Factors and Ergonomics Society, 2010. **52**(2): 295–307.

22. Reason, J., *Human error: Models and management.* BMJ, 2000. **320**: 768–770.

23. O'Daniel, M. and A. Rosenstein, *Professional communication and team collaboration,* in *Patient Safety and Quality: An evidence-based handbook for nurses,* R. Hughes, ed. 2008, Rockville, MD: Agency for Healthcare Research and Quality.

24. Wilson, K.A., et al., *Errors in the heat of battle: Taking a closer look at shared cognition breakdowns through teamwork.* Human Factors: The Journal of the Human Factors and Ergonomics Society, 2007. **49**(2): 243–256.

25. Miller, A., et al., *Care coordination in intensive care units: Communicating across information spaces.* Human Factors: The Journal of the Human Factors and Ergonomics Society, 2010. **52**(2): 147–161.

26. Johnson, D. and F. Johnson, *Joining Together.* 10th ed. 2010, New Jersey: Pearson.

27. Youngberg, B., ed. *Patient Safety Handbook.* 2nd ed. 2013, Maryland: Jones & Bartlett Learning.

28. *Pathways for Patient Safety,* 2008, Higher Research & Education Trust, Institute for Safe Medication Practices, MGMA Centre for Research.

29. Salas, E., N. Cooke, and M. Rosen, *On teams, teamwork, and team performance: Discoveries and developments.* Human Factors, 2008. **50**(3): 540–547.

30. Yang, L., C. Huang, and K. Wu, *The association among project manager's leadership style, teamwork and project success.* International Journal of Project Management, 2011. **29**(3): 258–267.

31. Reynard, J., J. Reynolds, and P. Stevenson, *Practical Patient Safety,* 2009, Oxford: Oxford University Press.

32. Firth-Cozens, J., *Cultures for improving patient safety through learning.* Quality and Safety in Health Care, 2001. **10**: ii26–ii31.
33. Leonard, M., S. Graham, and D. Bonacum, *The human factor: The critical importance of effective teamwork and communication in providing safe care.* Quality and Safety in Health Care, 2004. **13**: 85–90.
34. McQueen, M., *The New Rules of Engagement: A guide to understanding and connecting with generation Y.* 2nd ed. 2011, Sydney: Nexgen Group.
35. Schuster, P. and L. Nykolyn, *Communication for Nurses,* 2010, Philadelphia: F.A. Davis.
36. Coiera, E. and V. Tombs, *Communication behaviours in a hospital setting.* BMJ, 1998. **316**: 673–676.
37. Wertz, A., et al., *Effects of sleep inertia on cognition.* JAMA, 2006. **295**: 163–164.
38. Gorman, J.C., N.J. Cooke, and E. Salas, *Preface to the Special Issue on Collaboration, Coordination, and Adaptation in Complex Sociotechnical Settings.* Human Factors: The Journal of the Human Factors and Ergonomics Society, 2010. **52**(2): 143–146.
39. Haig, K., S. Sutton, and J. Whittington, *SBAR: A shared mental model for improving communication between clinicians.* Journal on Quality and Patient Safety, 2006. **32**(3): 167–175.
40. Reason, J., *The Human Contribution: Unsafe acts, accidents and heroic recoveries,* 2008, Farnham, Surrey: Ashgate Publishing.
41. Salas, E., et al., *Team training in the skies: Does Crew Resource Management (CRM) training work?* Human Factors: The Journal of the Human Factors and Ergonomics Society, 2001. **43**(4): 641–674.
42. *Formalized communication between rural home health agency nurses and physicians leads to increased use of home health servcies, fewer inpatient admissions* [accessed 28 November 2011]. Available from: www.innovations.ahrq.gov/content.aspx?id=2067.
43. *The OSSIE Guide to Clinical Handover Improvement,* 2010, Sydney: Australian Commission on Safety and Quality in Health Care.
44. Friesen, M., S. White, and J. Byers, *Handoffs: Implications for nurses,* in *Patient Safety and Quality: An evidence-based handbook for nurses,* R. Hughes, ed. 2008, Rockville, MD: Agency for Healthcare Research and Quality.
45. *Joint Commission Patient Safety Goals for 2008,* VA National Center for Patient Safety.
46. *Patient Safety Solutions: Communication during patient handovers,* 2007, Geneva: World Health Organization.

6

Managing Risk – Learning From Errors

Introduction

The increasing focus on patient safety has led to a greater emphasis on managing the risk of errors and adverse events occurring. To do this an organisation needs a risk management process that identifies the risks, assesses the likelihood of the risk happening and the possible severity of consequences, and then seeks to reduce or eliminate the risk. One method of gathering data to inform risk management assessment is to use information gained by reviewing adverse events. This has led to a rise in adverse incident reporting systems. However, we know that these capture only a fraction of the incidents that occur [1, 2]. In the main the serious or catastrophic errors of commission are reported but those incidents that staff perceive to be less important, and errors of omission, are under-reported [1, 2]. The real value of the systems lies in the analysis of the reports, as these can help to identify factors that led to the incident and from there the development of strategies to prevent or minimise the errors in the future [3]. However, we know from research that the analysis of incidents and the reporting back to individuals involved in them is not done well [4].

This chapter begins with a brief overview of risk management and then focuses on the role of individual health practitioners in recognising and reporting adverse events and near misses; methods of investigating adverse events concentrating on system factors rather than individuals; and the importance of sharing lessons from adverse event reports. Before proceeding you may wish to review the description of adverse events, errors and near misses given in Chapter 1.

Risk Management

Risk management is a process whereby organisations identify, prioritise and address business and clinical risks [5, 6]. The management of risk can be reactive, where an organisation is reacting to errors and learning from them, or proactive, in which an organisation is using information from sources such as patient safety alerts, healthcare failures and coroners' courts to prevent errors occurring [4]. Risk management involves several key elements including:

- identifying risk using existing data on incidents within the organisation and by reviewing and assessing service delivery information from external sources
- analysing the risks to understand the causes and consequences (both quantitatively and qualitatively)
- prioritising the risks by assessing the likelihood of the identified risk occurring and the consequences if it does
- treating the risk by making decisions about how to control risks by preventing or reducing the chance of a risk event occurring and acting to minimise the consequences [5].

In the following section we are focusing on the reactive process of detecting adverse events and learning from them to improve patient care.

Recognising and Reporting Adverse Events and Errors

Humans often learn by making mistakes, that is, if they take the time to think about why the mistake happened, and what they can do to prevent the same thing happening in the future. For example, if I am driving into my garage in my car and I clip the wing mirror as I go in, not only am I cross that my car is damaged, I am also very keen to ensure it doesn't happen again! So I think about what may have contributed to the incident – I was in a hurry as I was late, and the rubbish bin was in a different place, and I swung around it, rather than getting out and moving it. I was also distracted by a discussion I was having with my daughter about why I will not allow her out socially on a school night and finally, I had a headache because I had not had time to stop for lunch and I was hungry and dehydrated. All of these things meant I was not concentrating in the same way and the result was a damaged car. To avoid this happening again I need to be more aware that when I am distracted, tired, hungry and in a hurry I am less likely to take the time to move the rubbish bin rather than try and drive around it!

In organisations the importance of learning from mistakes is magnified. Reynard et al. [7] describe safety improvements made by the Cleveland Railway Company in the 1930s. These improvements resulted from the processing of data from an accident and incident system, which was instituted to keep track of accidents. This was remarkable for the 1930s and one can only imagine how the workers felt about filling in the forms! What was even more remarkable for the times is the Railway Company not only collected the statistics about the incidents but also had a process of reviewing the data. The review of the data indicated that there were more accidents and incidents at one particular depot than all the others. When they investigated this they identified three factors that seemed to be contributing to the increased number of incidents. These were that a large proportion of the drivers were new and failed to recognise hazards on the road, there was a culture of casual attitudes to safety with some drivers and finally, some drivers had poor vision. Strategies were instituted to deal with all three factors, which led to a substantial reduction in accidents.

While this organisational learning from accidents and errors may not seem remarkable in today's climate, in the 1930s this was ground breaking. This is especially so considering that it is only since the pivotal 2000 IOM report [1], where adverse events and errors were measured objectively, that these were recognised as a problem in healthcare. Yet, intuitively it is obvious that humans were delivering healthcare and humans make mistakes, so many health practitioners will have known that adverse events, errors and near misses were happening. These would most likely have been dealt with at a local level, addressing the individuals involved. However, there was no appreciation that errors or adverse events could or should be recorded and/or investigated from an organisational perspective to contribute to collective system learning. A large part of this attitude related to the prevailing culture of perfection, where mistakes were viewed as aberrant or careless behaviour on the part of individuals [8].

On the whole we now appreciate that human behaviour is error prone, and it is organisational systems and processes that will help prevent errors rather than blaming and shaming individuals [9]. This understanding means that if we are to improve safety then we need to examine incidents whether they are adverse events, errors or near misses so that we can learn from them and improve organisation systems and processes. However, if incidents are to be examined then we need to know about them. This relies on an organisation having an effective system that records incidents, and on the people involved recognising the importance of reporting incidents.

There are many different types of systems for gathering accident and incident data. These systems may have voluntary or mandatory reporting, offer anonymity for the reporter, or require the person filing the report to be identified. The systems can have protected reporting which means they are confidential to the organisation but not anonymous, or they can be open access so the information can be accessed by all those in the organisation and also by individuals or external organisations [1, 10]. Regardless of the type, an effective incident system is one where the mechanism for filing reports is easy to access and intuitive to complete. In addition, the research indicates that a system where the investigation of the incident focuses on looking for the factors that contributed to the decisions and actions which led to the incident, rather than just on identifying individuals to 'blame and retrain', is more likely to be accepted and therefore used by health professionals [11, 12]. When health professionals are able to recognise that incident systems and resulting investigations are making a difference and leading to real improvements in patient safety they feel empowered and are more likely to report incidents [10, 13].

Health professionals are the key to reporting and learning from errors, and without their commitment and motivation to report accidents and errors any accident and incident system will be ineffective. Yet, there is considerable evidence that health professionals may be reluctant to report errors [12, 14, 15]. The reasons for this unwillingness include:

- uncertainty about how and what to report
- lack of understanding about why reporting is important
- too busy to report
- fear of disciplinary action or litigation
- lack of feedback or resulting corrective action
- system too complicated to use
- assumption that someone else will report
- perception that a lack of harm to the patient negates need to report [7, 16].

Also of note is that different professionals have different reporting rates, with nurses more likely than medical staff to report incidents [16]. This is possibly related to practitioners having dissimilar professional cultural norms, the hierarchical nature of healthcare teams and the fear of litigation [16].

Many of the barriers identified above can be attributed to the organisational culture. A positive organisational culture is one in which health practitioners feel comfortable highlighting areas of concern. When issues are raised they are investigated and feedback is provided to staff about the outcome and strategies to address the concerns. There is regular education and support for staff to learn about safety systems and patient safety [7]. To encourage staff to report incidents, organisations need to be clear about what constitutes an incident. It may be that the organisation only wants reports of incidents where there is an adverse outcome for patients, or there may be a list of sentinel events that must be reported if they happen. It may be that the organisation only wants near misses reported. Or it may be any combination of these types of events. However, it is clear that without some guidelines of what constitutes a reportable event the reporting will be patchy [16].

Individuals are influenced by the social climate, beliefs and values of those with whom they work [17]. The attitudes and behaviours of staff are crucial to fostering a culture that encourages reporting of incidents. For instance, if a student or new graduate is working in a team that does not value input or feedback they are very unlikely to report practices which they may recognise as deviating from the evidence based practices they have been taught. Conversely if they are working in a team which values feedback and learning from each other they are more likely to raise concerns about practices that they perceive may be outdated [16].

Strong leadership that is committed to patient safety is required if an organisation is going to be able to foster and grow a culture where staff are encouraged to raise areas of concern. The leadership and management team must be committed to putting in place systems and processes which support open and inclusive communication [8]. In addition, the system should not be punitive but rather foster a positive learning climate where incidents are investigated to identify contributing factors, and feedback about the process and improvements are communicated to staff in a timely manner [18].

If the barriers to reporting can be overcome then the next challenge for health professionals is recognising what should be reported. What can seem an everyday 'hiccup' in the process of patient care may in fact be a 'red flag' that in some situations will lead to an adverse event. For example, imagine a busy operating theatre suite (OT) where there are 10 theatres working every day for 12 hours. In this OT the theatre staff for each of the theatres check in the patients for their allocated theatre. It is not unusual for a patient to be brought to OT with incorrect identification, consent forms not signed, the surgical site not being marked or current test results not being available in the notes. However, because many different staff are involved each day in checking patients into the OT, over time any one staff member may only encounter the problem infrequently. As each individual staff member encounters the problem for the particular patient they are checking in they rectify the problem by finding an instant solution. No harm is done and so there is no accident or incident report generated. Although the staff may all grumble about the problem in the tearoom, they accept these poor practices as 'just one of the things that is always happening around here' – this is called *normalisation of deviance* [10]. Nobody is aware of the frequency with which the problem is occurring, until one day there is a major incident involving wrong site surgery. The investigating team identifies that inadequate patient preparation for OT is widespread, leading to a situation when all the checks in the system failed and an adverse event occurred. If you review Reason's Swiss Cheese model in Chapter 1 you will see that this example fits this error model.

Reporting of incidents requires the individuals involved making a judgement about the 'worthiness' of the incident with regard to whether it should be reported or not. If there is an error with an obvious adverse outcome for the patient it is easy for the practitioner to recognise that this should be reported – for instance, a patient falls and suffers a subdural haemorrhage as a result. However, if the error does not lead to an adverse outcome for the patient, it is more likely that the practitioner may not see the value in reporting the incident [10] – a 'no harm done' approach. This judgement is influenced by the experience of the practitioner, with the experienced practitioner being able to recognise the potential for a serious event from a near miss because of their previous experiences. Conversely, this experience can have the opposite effect as experienced practitioners are normalised to deviance (they have seen the same thing happen many times before and nothing bad happens) whereas a less experienced practitioner can question what is normal and can act as a stimulus to report an incident. The skill of anticipation is important here – the ability to think that something dreadful could occur if preventative processes are not put in place.

Exercise 6.1

Aim of the exercise: To identify the impediments for individuals reporting incidents.

What to do:

1. Read the case studies presented here and consider the questions that follow.

Case Study 1

Shaftesbury ward was a very busy surgical ward with a rapid turnover and many complex care cases. David (22) was a first year general nursing student. He was an enthusiastic learner with great promise and seemed mature beyond his years. On this hectic Wednesday morning shift David was assigned to work in the RED team with six preoperative patients. As the surgery schedule was moving along quicker than anticipated, the surgical unit phoned the ward asking for the next patient – Mr Rambuku. Rosemary the ward clerk took the phone message and verbally passed it on to Sheena the charge nurse and Zoe the RED team leader. This unexpected request added to the hubbub on the ward. Zoe approached David and asked him to check the pre-medication against the sheet. All seemed in order so Zoe gave the pre-med to Mr Rambuku but when she went to sign the sheet it had already been signed by Sheena who had given the medication to help speed things along. Once the error had been recognised it was reported to the surgical team who monitored the patient until the effects of the overdose of pre-med wore off. The patient then went on to have his surgery with no complications and made an excellent recovery. As there were no ill-effects of the medication the decision was taken that an incident form did not need to be completed.

Case Study 2

Coleen worked in the administrative section of the hospital and got on really well with her boss Colin who was responsible for financial planning and managing. The section was a really great place to work with a supportive team spirit across the group. A few weeks after the end of the financial planning and approval process Coleen found a real error in the data which meant that more funds (over $500,000) would be attributed to the administrative section and diverted away from direct clinical services in aged care.

Coleen did not know what to do. She checked and re-checked the data but the error remained steadfast. If she raised the error it would undermine Colin's position and she did not wish to do this as he was such a good boss. But if the error was not corrected then old people might receive poor care resulting from diminished resources. It was not her mistake. It was unlikely that anybody would notice as the budget had already been approved ... She let it go.

2. Should both of these incidents be reported considering only one resulted in any direct patient effect? If so why, and if not why not?
3. What factors may have discouraged the people involved from reporting these incidents?
4. What factors would encourage the people involved to report these incidents in the future?
5. Discuss your findings with colleagues and in doing so identify how you could apply this type of situation to your own workplace.
6. Compare your findings with the Exercise Feedback section at the end of the chapter.

So far in this chapter we have focused on the organisational and system requirements for recognising and reporting incidents. However, you may find that you are working in an organisation where the guidelines for reportable incidents are not clear, yet in your daily work you encounter near miss incidents, errors and adverse events. How will you make the decision about which should be reported? While there is no absolute framework for you as an individual to make a decision about reportable or non-reportable events, in the absence of organisational guidelines we would suggest that the CUS tool (Concerned, Uncomfortable, Safety Issue) discussed in Chapter 5 may provide you with some guidance. If you as an individual practitioner recognise a near miss incident, an error or an adverse event you should ask yourself:

- Are you **concerned** about the incident?
- Are you **uncomfortable** about the incident?

If the answer to both of these questions is yes then this is a **safety issue** and should be reported. At the very least these issues need to be processed within the group or team so that all of the relevant aspects of the near miss can be identified in a clear and objective manner. This will help to ensure that a good decision is made.

To improve patient safety, then, requires that individuals recognise and report incidents, and that organisations have an effective reporting system and a culture that encourages reporting [19]. However, capturing the data about accidents and incidents within an organisation will not automatically lead to improvement in patient safety. Achieving improvement requires investigation of the factors that led to a specific event as well as examining the data to look for trends that may indicate an overall system problem. In the next section we will look at several methods of investigating single incidents. We will then look at the value of exploring recurring patterns in data and sharing this information to improve patient safety.

Investigation of Incidents

A health organisation will have many incident reports, many near misses (which may not be documented) and a large body of external reports that could be chosen as a focus of review. So, there is a need to have some scheme for prioritising those incidents that are going to be the focus of a formalised investigation and those that will be recorded and analysed as part of trending data. Runciman et al. [18] provide some guidance for prioritising the decision on incident investigation:

1. Problems that are common or routinely consume resources (e.g. poor adherence to protocols or policies)
2. Rare but dangerous events (e.g. two different doses of the same drug on a resuscitation trolley)
3. Events with an abhorrent outcome (e.g. incorrect cross match transplanted organs leading to death of recipient)
4. Topical issues (e.g. poorly sterilised instruments leading to HIV infections in patients) [18: 257].

Prioritisation may also be guided by the impact or harm that resulted from the incident. The NHS uses terms that grade the incidents from 'no harm' through low, moderate, severe and death. The system adopted by many of the states in Australia is similar, with a numerical rating being given to each incident based on the level of risk and the severity of the outcome associated with the incident [4].

Conventionally when incidents and adverse events are examined the focus is on seeking answers to what happened, how it happened, why it happened and what can be learnt in order to prevent similar incidents happening again. However, a very real difficulty in incident investigation is a tendency to label the cause of the error as human error, that is to say that the incident wouldn't have happened if those at the sharp end had not made a mistake. Think back to the discussion in Chapter 1 which highlighted human factors and slips, lapses, mistakes and violations that result in errors in patient care. These errors are called active errors as they occur at the interface between the health professional and the patient in the care process. It is important to identify the active errors that were involved in the incident being investigated as there may be deficits of skill or knowledge that need to be addressed. However, any strategies that are put in place to address an individual's performance may prevent that person making a similar error but are unlikely to stop the next person in a similar situation making the same type of error. An investigation that focuses purely on the active failure that contributed to the incident and ignores the work environment, the management processes and the organisational context is flawed and misses the opportunity to identify the latent factors that influence staff performance and lead to errors [20].

The principle underpinning a good investigation of an error is not to find out what people did wrong but rather to try and understand why, at the time, the decisions that were made seemed logical and the right thing to do. Unfortunately this is not as easy as it may sound, since looking back at a situation, once it is over, gives us a much better overview of the choices and actions that seem obviously the right thing to have done. This phenomenon is called hindsight bias and is very difficult for us to avoid in daily life, let alone when investigating an incident which had a poor outcome. The problem with hindsight bias is that knowing the outcome automatically colours our perception of the players' actions and decision making, because we can see that what they did led to the incident [21]. After the event we have access to a wider overview of the situation. We have access to critical information and knowledge including knowing what the outcome was, whereas the players at the time will only have knowledge of the immediate situation. This tends to make us judge the people, their actions and the processes in a negative way without understanding the complexity of the event [21–23].

As an example, think about all those times when our favourite sporting team loses an important game. Imagine we are watching the replay on TV; we can see exactly where the players went wrong, and missed opportunities to score or to block the other team scoring. Unfortunately, the players on the ground at the time couldn't see everything that was going on and could only make choices about the play based on what was happening immediately in front of them.

It is important then, in any incident investigation, to avoid a narrow focus on active errors at the sharp end, and to be aware of the dangers of hindsight bias. A successful incident investigation will involve techniques that allow the investigators to 'dig' deeper into the event to identify the 'what, how and why'. There are several formalised methods of analysing events that can be employed:

- Root cause analysis is a deliberate comprehensive dissection of the error looking for underlying causes.
- London Protocol, also known as cause analysis, is based on root cause analysis but is a less intense, structured process of reflection on an incident.
- Failure mode analysis is a proactive process to identify the likelihood that a particular piece of equipment or system process will fail.
- Barrier analysis is a technique often used particularly in process industries. It is based on tracing energy flows, with a focus on barriers to those flows, to identify how and why the barriers did not prevent the energy flows from causing harm.
- Change analysis is an investigation technique often used for problems or accidents. It is based on comparing a situation that does not exhibit the problem to one that does, in order to identify the changes or differences that might explain why the problem occurred.
- Causal factor tree analysis is a technique based on displaying causal factors in a tree-structure such that cause–effect dependencies are clearly identified. [4, 8, 24–27]

We will not examine all of these processes in depth, as further information is available in the references, but we will review the process of root cause analysis. This is used extensively across the world and illustrates the important process and depth of inquiry which can inform any incident investigation [28].

Root Cause Analysis

Root cause analysis (RCA) is based on the principle that it is necessary to understand both the active and latent failures as factors that lead to an incident. An important feature of root cause analysis is that it aims improvement strategies at root causes as this is more effective than merely treating the symptoms of the problem [29]. To be effective, a RCA must be performed systematically, and conclusions must be backed up by evidence, and there is usually more than one root cause for any given problem.

General process for performing root cause analysis

1. Define the problem
2. Gather data/evidence
3. Identify issues
4. Find root causes
5. Develop solution recommendations
6. Implement the recommendations
7. Observe the recommended solutions to ensure effectiveness.

The investigating team should be multidisciplinary and should gather together to examine the data and evidence in a systematic way. The data and evidence net needs to be spread wide in order to gather all the relevant information that will shed light on the root cause of the incident. This may include a review of medical records and other documentation relevant to the context (rosters, procedural manuals, etc.), interviews, and witness statements.

The role of the investigating team is to get to the root cause by asking the question 'why?' By repeatedly asking the question 'why' (five is a good rule of thumb), it is possible to peel away the layers of symptoms, which can lead to the root cause of a problem. Very often the ostensible reason for a problem will lead you to another question. For example:

1. *Why did the patient get the wrong dose of medication? The answer: Because the nurse administered the wrong dose of medication.*

In an RCA investigation the next question would be:

2. *Why did the nurse administer the wrong dose of medication? The answer: Because the medication comes in two different dosages*

– 5 mg and 10 mg – the nurse gave 10 mg when the dose prescribed was 5 mg.

The next question might be:

3. *Why did the nurse not realise there were different dosages? The answer: Because commonly on this particular ward only one dosage (5 mg) is used and normally that is all there is available on the ward. At this particular time there was a patient receiving 10 mg so both dosages were on the ward.*

The next question might be:

4. *Why did the nurse not notice that she was dispensing from a 10 mg package when she was checking the drug for administration? Answer: The different dosages of the drug look similar and come in similar packaging. As she was administering the drugs she was interrupted by another staff member and therefore lost concentration. When she returned her attention to the administration she did not realise that she hadn't checked it properly.*

And so the questions could go on in this 'laddering' manner to elicit a richer account of how this incident came to pass. Exploring an incident in this way and engaging different people can generate both explicit and tacit knowledge. Hopefully this example has served to illustrate that there can be many latent factors contributing to the actual error of the wrong dosage of medication. If you review Chapter 3 you should be able to identify several of the common latent factors, and if we continued the 'why' questioning there may well be a few more.

There may be many and varied contributing causes to any one incident. The following list gives some factors that should be considered in an RCA:

- institutional factors
- organisational and management factors
- work environmental factors
- team factors
- individual factors
- task factors
- patient factors [25, 29].

Root cause analysis is a time consuming and resource intensive process, and thus is not suitable for the investigation of all events. However, the process of RCA allows for a systematic investigation, which goes beyond the level of blaming individuals by focusing on system and process failures that have allowed the error to occur. Once the causes have been identified then a decision needs to be taken about strategies to manage the underlying causes to minimise the risk of the error happening again.

Although RCA is recognised as an important tool in the investigation of incidents, there are several limitations and barriers to its effective use. The major limitation is that a thorough RCA is time consuming and resource intensive. Additionally, the investigation team must all be trained in the process and understand the clinical and organisational context. Many teams report that the implementation of the recommendations that arise from an RCA are often not followed up or fully actioned. The literature reports that investigation teams commonly find they face the barriers of lack of time and resources, uncooperative colleagues, difficulty with teams and unsupportive management [29–33]. These factors can undermine the effectiveness of RCA and any other formal methods used for analysing incidents.

Exercise 6.2

Aim of the exercise: To practise using different methods of accident and incident investigation.

What to do:

1. Read the following case study and then answer the questions.

    A patient went to the operating room (OR) for surgery on the lower leg. Per the Universal Protocol, the surgeon marked the proper leg prior to bringing the patient to the OR. The patient was placed in the prone position and anesthesia was administered. A 'Time Out' was performed, during which all the team members met and confirmed the procedure. The nurse began to prep the patient's lower leg, but the anesthesiologist felt that something wasn't right. After stabilizing the patient, he checked the chart and discovered that the nurse had scrubbed the wrong extremity. He notified the team members and stopped the procedure. The patient had come just minutes away from having surgery on the wrong leg, but no harm occurred. The correct leg was then prepared, and the patient underwent successful surgery.

2. Imagine that you are a member of the investigating team. What barriers to the investigation might you encounter?
3. Using your knowledge of healthcare undertake an analysis of the incident using the root cause analysis methodology. You need to make some assumptions about the contributing factors, but you should formally write questions and answers using the 'five why' as demonstrated in the section above.
4. Make recommendations to prevent similar incidents happening again.
5. Discuss and compare your findings with colleagues.
6. Compare your findings with the Exercise Feedback section at the end of the chapter.

In spite of the recognised limitations and barriers to RCA, recommendations from RCA can be effective in changing practice to improve patient safety within the organisation or department in which the incident occurred. However, learning from incidents should also be available to the wider context of healthcare. In the next section we will focus on sharing lessons from adverse events.

Sharing Lessons from Adverse Events

Latent organisational factors that lead to an error in one healthcare context are likely to present in other contexts as well. The incidents involving injections of the chemotherapy agent Vincristine being administered intrathecally (via the spinal route) rather than intravenously, with disastrous results for patients, provide an excellent example of this. These incidents were occurring worldwide, and it was the sharing of information about them that resulted in recognition of common factors and the adoption across different organisations and countries of strategies to prevent similar tragedies [7]. Thus, although investigating single incidents to identify contributing active and latent failures is important, so also is trending the information from incidents within an organisation and sharing the information outside that organisation.

Many countries have national or system wide adverse event reporting systems. The National Reporting and Learning System (NRLS), which is in place in the NHS in the UK, is an example of a national system. This system requires incidents to be reported onto a national database by staff at a local level. The data is then analysed for trends and patterns and is used to develop strategies to improve patient safety [34]. Alerts and information are disseminated to NHS organisations by a tiered system, involving three levels of implementation advice. A *safety alert* requires prompt action by organisations to address high risk problems, a *safer practice notice* strongly advises implementation of a particular recommendation, and a *patient safety information alert* recommends that the information should be contemplated to improve patient safety [3].

Major catastrophic adverse events are often captured by the requirement to report sentinel events to health authorities or regulatory bodies. This system is in place in Australia and in the US. In Australia sentinel events include retained instruments after surgery, haemolytic blood transfusion reactions, maternal death, and infant discharge to the wrong family. In the US sentinel events include surgery on the wrong person and inpatient suicide. Both countries also include an 'other' category where organisations can report any other clinical catastrophic event that might occur. The reports are then reviewed by a panel of experts with a focus on the possibility that the event could occur in other organisations given a similar set of circumstances [4].

It must be noted that although the value in learning from errors, near misses and adverse events to improve patient safety is enormous, this is a reactive strategy. Organisations can also utilise proactive risk management approaches by putting prevention strategies in place to avoid errors before they occur. Sources that inform these proactive strategies include reports from coroners' inquests, commercial requirements to report adverse events (drug reactions, equipment problems), media reports, articles and reports in professional journals and health inquiries. The value of this type of information is enormous, with health organisations being able to learn from a much larger collection of adverse events than may occur or be reported within a single organisation [1].

Exercise 6.3

Aim of the exercise: To identify some different sources of information about adverse events.

What to do:

1. Access and read at least three of the resources below and address the questions.

   - www.nrls.npsa.nhs.uk/alerts/
   - www.safetyandquality.gov.au/internet/safety/publishing.nsf/Content/NIMC_005_Medication-Safety-Alerts
   - www.safetyandquality.health.wa.gov.au/home/patient_news.cfm
   - https://www.ecri.org/PatientSafety/Pages/WHO_Patient_Safety_Alerts.aspx
   - www.fda.gov/Safety/MedWatch/SafetyInformation/default.htm

2. Choose two alerts that may be applicable in the area of health in which you work or are familiar with. Are you aware that these alerts have been identified within the health organisation?
3. Identify strategies you could utilise to disseminate the information about the alerts in the workplace.
4. Discuss your findings with colleagues.
5. Compare your findings with the Exercise Feedback section at the end of the chapter.

Summary

In this chapter we focused on the importance of recognising and reporting adverse events, the investigation of incidents and the sharing of information to learn from incidents. We examined one incident investigation tool called root cause analysis in some depth to demonstrate the need to identify both active and latent factors contributing to errors. Analysis of this nature is often a prerequisite for improving patient safety.

In the next chapter we will be exploring the human side of safe work practice. We will bring together the information and lessons learnt in previous chapters and use them as a basis for providing techniques for individual practitioners to develop situational awareness in their everyday practice and in crisis situations.

The themes of this chapter relate to the WHO curriculum guideline topics of [35]:

- Learning from errors to prevent harm
- Understanding and managing clinical risk.

The Exercise Feedback below provides an overview of the key points of this chapter.

EXERCISE FEEDBACK

Exercise 6.1

Both of the incidents described in these case studies should be reported. Even though one scenario did not result in any direct patient effect, without knowledge of the error there is no way the organisation can identify where the system broke down and how these shortfalls allowed the error to occur. Once the system problem is identified the organisation is in a position to put strategies in place to prevent the error occurring again.

The factors that discourage people reporting errors include:

- uncertainty about how and what to report
- lack of understanding about why reporting is important
- too busy to report
- fear of disciplinary action or litigation
- lack of feedback or resulting corrective action
- system too complicated to use
- assumption that someone else will report
- perception that lack of harm to the patient negates need to report
- lack of professional attitudes and values
- burnout at work.

Practitioners are more likely to report incidents in an organisational culture where they feel comfortable reporting incidents, where they can see that incidents are investigated and feedback is provided, and where they can see that strategies are instigated to prevent the recurrence of the incident.

Exercise 6.2

Effective RCAs are time consuming and resource intensive. The barriers that RCA teams often face are a lack of time and resources, as well as uncooperative colleagues, difficulty with teams and unsupportive management.

Although one question leads to another in the RCA process your questions would be focused around the flaws in the timeout process. The factors you should be considering when formulating the questions should include the following:

- institutional factors
- organisational and management factors
- work environmental factors
- team factors
- individual factors
- task factors.

Your recommendations should focus on system improvements rather than on any one individual's performance. In making the recommendations you should include a process of monitoring and review to ensure that recommendations are implemented and evaluated for effectiveness in terms of improving the timeout process.

Exercise 6.3

Incident reporting systems and the subsequent process of investigating and instituting strategies to prevent a reoccurrence is important to improve patient safety. This process is a reactive process, that is, we wait for an incident to occur and then act to prevent it happening again. Exercise 6.3 aimed to highlight the fact that there are also proactive strategies which organisations can and should be using to prevent errors before they happen. Organisations can identify where there are risks by utilising sources such as reports from coroners' inquests, commercial requirements to report adverse events (drug reactions, equipment problems), media reports, articles and reports in professional journals and health inquiries.

References

1.   IOM, *To Err is Human: Building a safer health care system*, 2000, Washington, DC: National Academy Press.

2. Leape, L. and D. Berwick, *Five years after To Err is Human: What have we learnt?* JAMA, 2005. **293**: 2384–2390.
3. Milligan, F., *Implementing solutions to prevent patient harm.* Nursing Standard, 2006. **20**(19): 56–59.
4. Wolff, A. and S. Taylor, *Enhancing Patient Safety: A practical guide to improving quality and safety in hospitals*, 2009, Sydney: MJA Books.
5. Walshe, K., *The development of clinical risk management*, in *Clinical Risk Managment: Enhancing patient safety*, C. Vincent, ed. 2001, London: BMJ Books: 45–60.
6. Vincent, C., ed. *Clinical Risk Management: Enhancing patient safety.* 2nd ed. 2001, London: BMJ Books.
7. Reynard, J., J. Reynolds, and P. Stevenson, *Practical Patient Safety*, 2009, Oxford: Oxford University Press.
8. Wachter, R., *Understanding Patient Safety.* 2nd ed. 2012, San Francisco: McGraw-Hill.
9. Reason, J., *Human Error: Models and management.* BMJ, 2000. **320**: 768–770.
10. Davies, E. and P. Cleary, *Hearing the patient's voice? Factors affecting the use of patient survey data in quality improvement.* Quality and Safety in Health Care, 2005. **14**: 428–432.
11. Firth-Cozens, J., *Cultures for improving patient safety through learning.* Quality and Safety in Health Care, 2001. **10**: ii26–ii31.
12. Braithwaite, J., et al., *Cultural and associated enablers of, and barriers to, adverse incident reporting.* Quality and Safety in Health Care, 2010. **19**(3): 229–233.
13. Sitaru, D., *Corporate governance.* Lex ET Scientia, Juridical Series, 2009. **2**: 186–212.
14. Braithwaite, J., M. Westbrook, and J. Travaglia, *Attitudes toward the large-scale implementation of an incident reporting system.* International Journal for Quality in Health Care, 2008. **20**(3): 184–191.
15. Coulter, A., *Patients' expectations*, in *Medical Education and Training: From theory to delivery*, Y. Carter and N. Jackson, eds. 2009, Oxford: Oxford University Press: 45–57.
16. Kingston, M., et al., *Attitudes of doctors and nurses towards incident reporting: A qualitative analysis.* MJA, 2004. **181**(1): 36–39.
17. *Patient-centred Care: Improving quality and safety by focusing care on patients and consumers – Discussion Paper*, 2010, Australian Commission on Quality and Safety in Health Care.
18. Runciman, W., A. Merry, and M. Walton, *Safety and Ethics in Healthcare: A guide to getting it right*, 2007, Aldershot, Hampshire: Ashgate Publishing.
19. Shaw, J. and M. Baker, *"Expert patient" – dream or nightmare.* BMJ, 2004. **328**: 723.
20. Reason, J., J. Carthey, and M. de Leval, *Diagnosing "vulnerable system syndrome": An essential prerequisite to effective risk management.* Quality in Health Care, 2001. **10**: ii21–ii25.
21. Dekker, S., *Drift into Failure: From hunting broken components to understanding complex systems*, 2011, Farnham, Surrey: Ashgate Publishing.
22. Dekker, S., *Patient Safety: A human factors approach*, 2011, Boca Raton, Florida: CRC Press.
23. Woods, D., et al., *Behind Human Error*, 2010, Farnham, Surrey: Ashgate Publishing.

24. James, J., *A Sea of Broken Hearts*, 2007, Bloomingham: Authorhouse.
25. Hovey, R., et al., *Patient safety: A consumer's perspective*. Qualitative Health Research, 2011. **21**: 662–672.
26. Frampton, S. and P. Charmel, eds. *Putting Patients First: Best practices in patient-centred care*. 2nd ed. 2009, San Francisco: Jossey-Bass.
27. Reason, J., *Beyond the organisational accident: The need for "error wisdom" on the frontline*. Quality and Safety in Health Care, 2004. **13**: 28–33.
28. Edwards, M., *Public sector governance – Future issues for Australia*. Australian Journal of Public Administration, 2002. **61**(2): 51–61.
29. Feinman, J., *Why sorry doesn't need to be the hardest word*. BMJ, 2011. **342**: 1238–1239.
30. Boyle, S., *Impact of changes in organisational structure on selected key performance indicators for cultural organisations*. International Journal of Cultural Policy, 2007. **13**(3): 319–334.
31. Cartwright, J., et al., *Patient and Public Involvement Toolkit*, 2011, West Sussex: Wiley-Blackwell.
32. *Ontario Medical Association – Policy on Patient-Centred Care*, Ontario Medical Review, 2010. June: 34–49.
33. Lega, F., *Organisational design for health integrated delivery systems: Theory and practice*. Health Policy, 2007. **81**: 258–279.
34. *Seven Steps to Patient Safety: The full reference guide*, 2004, National Patient Safety Agenda, NHS.
35. *WHO Patient Safety Curriculum Guide: Multi-professional edition*, 2011, Geneva: World Health Organization.

7

Situation Awareness

Introduction

In this chapter we will explore the concept of situation awareness and the importance of this for patient safety. Throughout the book we have emphasised that blaming and shaming the individual when an error happens, and assuming that training or removing the individual from the sharp end will prevent future errors, is not the strategic solution to improving patient safety. Instead we have focused on system solutions where we look for the latent factors that may have created an error prone situation in which humans are more likely to make errors. Our understanding of how humans process information and then use this as a basis for taking actions (either consciously or unconsciously) underpins our knowledge of human fallibility. The study of human factors then uses this to inform the design of work systems, processes, technology and the work environment to reduce the risk of errors.

In this chapter the focus is more on the sharp end of the errors, and the individuals who work there. While acknowledging that system improvement using our knowledge of human factors is a vital component for improving patient safety, the other vital element required for improving patient safety is for individuals to be able to recognise error prone conditions and to be able to act appropriately to reduce the risk of error [1, 2]. This chapter brings together the information and lessons from previous chapters and uses them as a basis for developing tools and techniques to enhance situational awareness in everyday practice and in emergency situations. This will include further consideration of the cognitive processes involved in situational awareness (see Chapter 1 for a review of cognitive processes and error).

We will also discuss factors that can lead to the loss of situation awareness, which in turn provides insights into the strategies that will mitigate the risk of this happening. These strategies include organisational processes such as checklists, clinical simulation training and education. We will conclude with some discussion about techniques that individuals can utilise to recognise and manage personal stressors, the environmental context and the task being undertaken, all factors that can influence the development of situation awareness. We will begin the chapter by discussing the general concept of situation awareness, but first a short story:

> Imagine that it is very late on a dark, forbidding moonless night. You missed the last bus and you have to walk from the train station to your home, which is a mile away. The route you have to walk is down a long lane, with poor street lighting and very few houses. It is cold, windy, and lonely. Recently there have been several incidents of assaults in this particular area. You start walking towards home – all your senses are on high alert and you are listening for footsteps, you are straining to see in the night shadows to detect anything untoward. You are aware that this is a potentially hazardous situation, so you have your mobile in your hand ready to call for help, you are noting where the houses are that you could run to for help, and you are walking very quickly and avoiding where you can the dark shadows. You are aware and mindful of your situation and have contingencies in place to deal with the problem if it happens. You definitely have very high situation awareness! Contrast this with the situation the next day when you are walking back to the train station, the sun is shining and the morning is fine and warm. There are lots of people about and many smile at you and nod hello as you walk past. You stroll along, daydreaming about the weekend, hardly aware of your surroundings at all. In this situation you have low situation awareness.

What Do We Mean by the Term Situation Awareness?

> Two men look out through the same bars; one sees the mud, and one the stars. (Frederick Langbridge, 1849–1923)

Throughout our day-to-day activities we are constantly processing information about what is going on around us and making sense of this information so that we can carry out tasks, make decisions and generally just function normally as a human being in our surroundings. However, depending on circumstances we are more or less aware of how we are handling and processing the information about our current situation. In novel, acute or serious situations, we tend to have a high degree of awareness of our surroundings. This is described as situation awareness. The non-technical description of situation awareness is 'knowing what is going on'. The technical definition of situation awareness is 'the *perception* of elements in relation to time and space, *comprehension* of their meaning, and *projection* into the near future' [3: 202].

Situation awareness requires all three elements of perception, comprehension and projection. Perception is the process of monitoring and noticing what is going on around us by recognising the features of our surroundings – this could include objects, people, events, environmental context – and noting their current status. Comprehension involves identifying how the information we perceive around us fits together and making sense of it. Projection involves using our perceptions and comprehension about the situation to make assumptions about what will or may happen next [3–5]. We call this forming a mental model of a given situation. People use these mental models of a situation as a basis for decisions about future actions [6]. You will remember that we discussed shared mental models in Chapter 5 in relation to teamwork and communication. Effective teamwork occurs when people share a similar perception, comprehension and projection of a given situation [7]. Flawed mental models based on incorrect perceptions, comprehension and projections result in poor or wrong decisions and incorrect actions taken in a given situation.

Exercise 7.1

Aim of the exercise: To consider the development of mental models.

What to do:

1. Read the following scenario and then answer the questions.

    Tara (38) is married to Ben (42), a local fireman. They are conscientious and loving parents with two children – Cassandra (4) and Daniel (2). Last night Tara went out on the town with her girlfriends, one of whom was celebrating her fortieth birthday. She drank a lot of wine and came home quite drunk. She arranged with Ben to sleep in late while he looked after the children that morning. As it happened Ben was unexpectedly called into work following a major accident on the freeway. After securing the stair gate and seeing that the children were playing happily in their bedroom Ben left for work. Tara was still pretty groggy and lay on her bed in a drowsy state but she could hear the children in the next room.

    She woke to Cassandra's shrieking cries, jumped off the bed and stood at the top of stairs. At the bottom of the stairs Daniel lay motionless with a bloodied face. Cassandra was very distressed as she told Tara how Daniel had forced the stair gate and fallen head first down the stairs. Daniel recovered quickly and all three went to the local Emergency Department for a check up. Checks revealed that Daniel had sustained no serious injury apart from a small cut on his forehead.

However, Beverly – the junior doctor who examined Daniel – was very concerned about his welfare and saw an unsupervised, injured child who arrived in the department with a mother reeking of alcohol. She commented to her colleagues how alcoholism is a major risk factor and asked if they had noticed anything worrisome with Daniel or Cassandra. Mary (the nurse in charge) knew both Tara and Ben very well and reassured Beverly that this was a very unusual set of circumstances. However, Beverly was not convinced and asked to check the family health records for other accidents or injuries. Although there were no other recorded incidents Beverly still insisted that the family be reported for follow-up investigation by the social worker.

2. Make some notes about the information you think Beverly is basing her mental model on.
3. Now think about a similar situation, but imagine that Tara did not smell of alcohol when she presented with Daniel. Do you think this might have resulted in a different mental model being developed by Beverly? If so why, and if not why not?
4. Identify from your own practice environment where inaccurate mental models could compromise patient safety.
5. Discuss and compare your findings with colleagues. Are there particular things that stand out from your discussions that have relevance for how inaccurate mental models can impact on patient safety?
6. Compare your findings with the Exercise Feedback section at the end of the chapter.

What Affects Situation Awareness?

Formation of an accurate mental model of a given situation relies on an individual's internal processes of perception, comprehension and projection. However, this internal processing is affected by several factors, including the individual's cognition processes, the individual's knowledge, experience and current personal stress factors, the task being undertaken in terms of complexity and familiarity, and the environmental context in which the person is working [8]. Figure 7.1 illustrates the relationship of these factors.

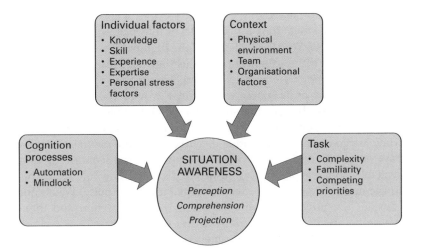

Figure 7.1 Factors affecting an individual's situation awareness

The lack or loss of situation awareness in a given situation is influenced by these four factors, which can result in flawed processes of perception, comprehension or projection, leading to an inaccurate mental model. This then leads to erroneous decisions and actions arising from the inaccurate mental model. We will now discuss each of these in turn. You will note that more time is spent on cognition processes. This is not because they are more important but rather that their influence on situation awareness may be more of a novel concept to many and thus more involved to explain.

Cognition Processes

In a complex situation the way our attention is focused will influence how cues in the environment around us are processed. This processing involves delving into our memories and matching patterns with what we have already experienced or know. An example of this is when we take a patient's pulse. If the pulse is 140 beats per minute, and we had had experience nursing paediatric patients, we would not be worried if this was an infant as this rate is within normal range. However, if this was an adult and we were experienced adult nurses we would be aware that this pulse rate is high and would be looking for a reason for it. It may be that the person has just run up the stairs, or they have a fever, or there may be other reasons. Using our previous skills, knowledge and experiences we would look for other bits of information to make sense of the high pulse. We may well dismiss the high pulse as being nothing to worry about if the patient then tells us they have just rushed up the stairs because they were anxious at being late for the appointment. We use the exercise and anxiety to explain the high pulse. This is our tendency, to take the first hypothesis for which two pieces of confirmatory evidence appear [6]. This can then lead to a situation of mindlock where we go on to interpret other data to confirm the mental model we have developed of the situation even when there is disconfirming data available. So if the person was flushed and sweaty we would relate this to the mental model of an exercise related increased pulse. We do not consider the possibility that the person has an infection and these symptoms are related to that rather than exercise.

We can also form an incorrect mental model of a situation when we see links between data that are not there. This is called the assumed connection effect [3]. An example of this would be a patient who presents with a past history of aggression related to alcohol intake and a mental illness. When this patient displays aggressive behaviour on presentation, and we can smell alcohol on his breath, our mental model is that this is aggressive behaviour related to the alcohol and the mental illness. We plan our care based on this assumption. However, subsequently it is identified that the patient has pneumonia and the aggressive behaviour is related to hypoxia (low oxygen concentration). The alcohol and the past history of a mental illness had absolutely no relation to the current aggressive episode yet the mental model we formed linked the two pieces of data. The clinical treatment and management of hypoxia is very different to the treatment and management of aggression related to alcohol and a mental disorder. The outcome for the patient being treated incorrectly could be at best a delayed recovery and at worst catastrophic.

How important we perceive the cues to be will also influence whether we prioritise certain cues over others based on previous experience or knowledge. The accuracy of the mental model we form of a given situation is dependent on pattern matching the cues with other mental models. If the cues are mismatched, misinterpreted or there is information missing then the mental model formed will be inaccurate. The decisions based on that mental model will be wrong [9]. For example, a new practitioner in intensive care had identified that when a patient with a endotracheal tube had excessive secretions it was appropriate to provide endotracheal suctioning. Faced with a situation where a patient suddenly deteriorated, with a falling oxygen saturation and a large amount of frothy secretions bubbling from the endotracheal tube, the practitioner immediately applied endotracheal suctioning only to find that this did not alleviate the situation but rather worsened it – the oxygen saturation continued to fall and the secretions increased. In this situation, the patient had developed pulmonary oedema and suctioning the endotracheal tube was the wrong strategy and was exacerbating the problem. The practitioner had matched the mental model formed from past experience of increased secretions and falling oxygen saturations to the solution of suctioning secretions to improve the patient's airway. Never having had the experience of caring for a patient with pulmonary oedema, the practitioner was unable to form the correct mental model to determine the appropriate action.

Expectations also affect perception and cognition. We see what we expect to see in a particular situation or environment [4]. Think back to Chapter 4 when we looked at medication errors. Common errors occurred when the same drug with different dosages, or different drugs with similar looking packaging or similar sounding names, are stored together. When we reach for a particular medication we expect to see the particular medication and we interpret the information on name, dosage and packaging in a way that confirms in our mind that the medication we have is the one we want, when in fact this may not be the case – many incident reports identify that adverse events as a result of medication errors are linked to confusion related to similar packaging or similar drug names [10].

Another area that affects how we form mental models is the process of automaticity [4, 11]. This occurs when we do things that are routine on 'autopilot'. This can be positive in that it reduces demands on our limited capacity of attention and allows us to multi-task. Think about the times you have driven home on a familiar route and not been aware when you arrived of having driven there. The problem with automaticity is that it can also cause us to disregard or not recognise novel stimuli and then not respond appropriately. Verbal checking procedures have been developed to combat this problem, but as they become a routine task that is carried out many times a day they themselves can become an automatic process for the people involved and discrepancies can be easily missed [12]. For example, one study reported that 77 per cent of incorrect blood component transfusions involved checking procedures which had been instigated to prevent such errors [12].

We need to be clear here that this is not about people making deliberate choices to form incorrect mental models – rather these patterns of cognitive processes are tendencies that we are all subject to. Understanding this gives us insight into why people make the choices they do in terms of actions and decisions about care. This understanding also helps us identify strategies that will increase the likelihood of forming a correct mental model. We will discuss these strategies later in the chapter. The important point to remember here is that these factors influence how we view and interpret what is happening in the world.

Context Factors

Individuals are also affected by the context in which they are working, and this can have an impact on our situation awareness. If we are working in an environment that is unfamiliar, cluttered, poorly lit, very noisy with lots of distractions or highly complex and busy, this will affect our ability to perform well which then affects our cognitive processes [11, 13]. This type of environment can affect our working memory by diminishing the effectiveness of information gathering and our ability to process the information. Individuals become disorganised in how they gather information from the situation, paying less attention to peripheral information. There is a tendency to make a decision about required actions without reviewing all the available information [14]. Consider a busy intensive care unit with a plethora of different technical monitoring and clinical equipment providing information about each patient. The audible alarms and displays provide a visual and auditory cacophony of stimulation to the staff. While these are important to alert staff to clinical variations that require attention this can actually result in data overload for them as they try to process all the information [14].

We rely on accurate data to feed our perception, comprehension and projection. In the context where we are working with incomplete or incorrect information such as the wrong patient notes, missing information in notes, or inaccurate test results this will likely lead to a flawed mental model of the situation [9]. Consider the situation where a resident of an aged care facility who suffers from dementia falls while walking to the bathroom. The carer notes that the resident is able to stand immediately and so the incident is not reported in the notes. Later in the day the resident becomes aggressive and uncooperative, and the decision is taken to increase their sedation. It is not until the next day when significant bruising of the left leg is noted and the resident is now unable to walk that an X-ray is ordered and a fractured hip is diagnosed. The lack of information in the notes about the fall resulted in the carers having an incorrect mental model of why the resident was aggressive and uncooperative, thinking it related to the dementia not to pain from the fracture.

When we discussed teamwork and communication in Chapter 5 we highlighted that the cornerstone of a successful team was effective coordination, cooperation and communication. The competencies required to achieve good teamwork included leadership, situation monitoring, mutual support, adaptability, shared mental model, communication, collective orientation and mutual trust [15]. These competencies all contribute to both the individual and the team processing the available context specific information and using this to assess needs and plan actions drawn from an accurate mental model of the situation. [16]. The well-known case of Elaine Bromiley who died as a result of a team error illustrates this (you can view a reconstruction of this at www.chfg.org/articles-films-guides/just-a-routine-operation-teaching-video). In this unfortunate case Elaine Bromiley was undergoing routine nasal surgery, but the anaesthetist was unable to intubate her. The patient's oxygen saturations fell to critical levels – even when a second anaesthetist arrived the intubation failed. The recognised emergency protocol for this situation is immediate tracheostomy. However, the team continued to focus on trying to intubate. One of the nursing staff provided the emergency tracheostomy set and another called the intensive care unit to alert them to the emergency, but neither of these actions was recognised by the medical staff. It was another 35 minutes before the procedure was abandoned. Elaine Bromiley suffered irreparable brain damage related to hypoxia and died two weeks later [17]. This case illustrates how lack of both team and individual situation awareness as a consequence of poor teamwork, with no one taking overall leadership, poor communication between the nursing staff and medical staff and a loss of collective orientation led to an inadequate mental model of the dire circumstances and resulted in a poor outcome for the patient and her family [18].

Individual Factors

Having identified some of the context factors, it is important to note that other individual factors can also compromise an individual's ability to perform at their best. These are closely aligned with the situational awareness outlined earlier and can influence the ways a person conceives a situation. Fatigue can be a significant factor affecting an individual's ability to develop and maintain adequate situation awareness, as it affects the ability to process information and form accurate mental models of the situation [19]. Fatigue can be the result of workload intensity or, conversely, too little activity. Humans perform at their best under conditions of moderate stress/workload, and perform less well in situations of particularly high or low stress or workload [11]. Fatigue can also be caused by physical and psychological effort, sleep deprivation or disturbances, the time of the day, and disruption of circadian rhythms [6]. These conditions of course describe the working conditions of many healthcare clinicians!

Other short-lived factors such as anxiety, mental workload, negative life events, stress and illness may all affect the individual [14]. These may result in decreased reaction times, slower decision making and increases in slips, lapses and mistakes [20]. In addition, cognitive slowing as a result of these factors impacts on the individual's ability to maintain situation awareness as the ability to collect and process information is compromised [6].

An individual's previous experience, skills and knowledge, as well as their current workload, impacts on their capacity to focus on, and manage, the cognitive attention required to maintain situational awareness [21, 22].

Task Factors

The impact of task factors on situational awareness is related to complexity and/or familiarity with the task(s) being undertaken. For tasks that the person is very familiar with, they are more likely to omit steps and less likely to notice these errors as they undertake them with a degree of automaticity. This can lead to a loss of situation awareness as they do not include the likelihood that they have made an error in their mental model of the situation [3, 13, 23]. Conversely, tasks that are particularly complex or unfamiliar to the person can also lead to a loss of situation awareness as the greater the informational loading for an individual the more likely that attention will be diverted from other aspects of the situation going on around them. The following incident illustrates this.

Mary was an experienced surgical RN working on a busy surgical ward and had been buddied with a graduate nurse who was having difficulties settling into the role as a registered nurse. One of the postoperative patients had had a vaginal hysterectomy and required a vaginal packing to be removed. The graduate RN was very keen to take out the pack. After Mary had gone through the nursing policy and the doctor's strict instructions thoroughly with her, the graduate RN went and performed the procedure. A while afterwards Mary was with the patient who became very distressed. On further questioning she revealed that the nurse who had taken the pack out had not worn gloves during the procedure. The subsequent review identified that Mary had mentioned the need for a 'clean' procedure as listed in the policy (which required gloves but was not an aseptic procedure), but the graduate nurse in her anxiety had heard the instruction that it was not an aseptic procedure, and not recalling that any procedure that involved body fluids required gloves formed the inaccurate mental model that no gloves were required for the procedure.

The four factors of cognition, context, individual and task that affect situation awareness and the development of an accurate mental model are not discrete but overlap and interact. There are strategies that can help minimise the impact of them and we will discuss these in the next section. However, first complete the following exercise.

Exercise 7.2

Aim of the exercise: To consider the factors that impact on an individual's capability to maintain situation awareness.

What to do:

1. Read the following case study and then answer the questions.

    A 17-month-old female infant in the paediatric intensive care unit (PICU) developed acute respiratory failure.

    While setting up the laryngoscope and endotracheal tube, the PICU physician gave a verbal order for atropine, etomidate, and rocuronium (drugs used in the procedure for intubation). Shortly thereafter, but prior to intubation, the infant acutely desaturated (oxygen levels dropped). The team realized the patient received the paralytic agent prematurely. She was immediately intubated without difficulty and her respiratory status was stabilized.

> *Upon review of the event, the team discovered that the nurse, who was new to the PICU, had not realized the medication was a paralytic agent and thus administered it before the intubation tray was ready, resulting in the infant's desaturation.*
>
> *In this case, a child suffered a hypoxic episode (low oxygen levels) because she was paralyzed prematurely during an urgent, but not emergent, intubation procedure.*
>
> Reprinted with permission of AHRQ WebM&M. Source: Weinger MB, Blike GT. Intubation mishap. AHRQ WebM&M [serial online]. September 2003. Available at: www.webmm.ahrq.gov/case.aspx?caseID=29.

2. Identify the flawed mental models that the PICU physician who gave the medication order and the nurse who gave the drug were using to make decisions about their actions.

3. Note the accurate mental model that leads to the correct actions by the team to remedy the situation. What factors may have contributed to positive situation awareness of the team?

4. Make a list of the cognitive, context, individual and task factors that may have impacted on this situation for the nurse.

5. Discuss your findings with colleagues and friends. In your discussions identify how you can apply what you have learnt from this exercise.

6. Compare your findings with the Exercise Feedback section at the end of the chapter.

How Do We Optimise the Likelihood of the Development of Accurate Situation Awareness?

In the previous sections we have identified that in highly complex, dynamic, time critical environments, in which decisions made by participants may have serious outcomes, a high degree of situation awareness is crucially important. Of course, the descriptors 'highly complex, dynamic and time critical' are a perfect fit for the healthcare environment. A lack of situation awareness results in errors and adverse events. Strategies to address the different factors – cognition, context, individual and task – that impinge on situation awareness have been developed, and we will consider some of these below.

Checklists and Checking Procedures

Checklists and checking procedures are one useful method to increase situation awareness. Checklists can provide a 'memory jog' for people to highlight deviations from the normal process, which may be so predictable and routine that it can be done automatically. Checklists can support cognitive processes in stressful or time critical situations or where there are frequent interruptions [24]. However, checklists and checking procedures are only effective if they are given full attention when being carried out, and there are protocols that detail how, when and who is to carry out a check [3]. Lack of mindfulness to the process of checking items on a checklist was dramatically recognised following several airline crashes in the 1980s where subsequent review of the voice recorder demonstrated poor compliance with take-off protocols [16].

There are several different sorts of checklists. One common type is a challenge and response checklist [3]. It is most effective when each person involved responds verbally to each checkpoint confirming the item or action. For instance, a checking protocol may require that before administering medication a nurse verbally checks with another nurse at the bedside the patient's name, the administration time, the dose, the route and the drug. Of course, if this is done in a cursory manner – with a degree of robotic behaviour – this will not help with focusing attention on the situation at hand.

A second checklist procedure is a point and call system. Using this, the first person points to the medical orders, the display or the control lever and the second person states what is seen. For instance, when setting up for a radiotherapy procedure the first person may ask what the oncologist prescription is, and then what the exposure settings are on the machine, and the second person will read them back. However, once again these types of checks need to be undertaken with full attention. In a paper on automaticity, Toft and Mascie-Taylor reported a radiotherapy incident where checks by three different staff members resulted in the same error of dosage 10 different times even though they were using a checklist [12].

A further type of checklist is where the steps of a specific procedure are listed to remind the team of the actions required and their sequence. This type of list is helpful in emergency and non-routine situations. An example is the steps of Advanced Life Support, which may be listed next to the resuscitation trolley as a cue for staff.

Another type of checking procedure involves a process of team briefing where the team gives attention to each different aspect of the situation and notes their interpretation of what is going on or what is expected to happen. This ensures that members of the team are more aware of what is going on around them rather than just focusing on their part of the procedure. As well, it provides an opportunity for team members to challenge actions if they do not fit in with their perception of the situation [25]. This type of checking procedure works best in non-emergency situations where there is time to discuss the different aspects of the situation. However, this technique can be modified so that the briefing is more formalised and has an element of challenge and response in the format.

The design of checklists is crucial to their success. Those without check-off provisions are more likely to result in the overlooking of essential items – checklists with check-off provisions have an error rate of 3 in 1000 while those without have an error rate of 1 in 100 [26]. Checklists that require the checker to state 'check' or 'ok' are susceptible to error as the checking becomes automatic. Those that require the checker to state what they are seeing, maybe the patient's name and date of birth or what the setting on the machine reads, are less prone to automaticity errors [9].

Checklists should be short. If the procedure requires a long list then it should be divided into sections [27]; the WHO safe surgery checklist is an example, with a check-in, time-out and sign-out section. Moreover, those involved in using the checklist must be familiar with the terms used and the process for which it is being employed [27]. Finally, checklists should be reviewed and revised frequently to ensure they remain valid. One such method of reviewing (and initially developing) these is simulation, and we move on to discuss this in the next section.

Simulation

Simulation offers health professionals experience in critical and non-critical situations and allows people to build up a 'bank' of experiences on which to base future mental models [5]. Simulated experiences can be simple role-play scenarios or simulated experiences utilising technological resources that can replicate a variety of situations and outcomes. In addition to developing skills and knowledge in certain simulated situations there is also the opportunity to experience variations of a situation and new outcomes. This increases people's abilities to manage and cope in novel situations, decreasing the cognitive load and stress when faced with the situations for real [5, 23, 28].

Research has demonstrated that individuals in simulations are readily able to become involved as if it were a real situation and act as they would do if it was real [29]. Simulation can include a range of modalities including verbal role-playing scenarios, interactive mannequins or devices and complex computer simulations that provide a virtual reality [30].

Simulation has been used in the airline industry for many years to assess pilots' skills, knowledge and performance in specific situations [31]. Simulation is becoming more common in healthcare but is still mainly confined to the areas of conceptual knowledge and technical skills [29]. However, with the growing appreciation that non-technical skills such as situation awareness, leadership and communication, and teamwork are as important as technical skills in patient safety, there has been an increasing use of simulation experiences in these areas, providing the opportunity to review, learn and assess these skills [32].

Assessing Individual Capacity to Maintain Situation Awareness

We know that humans are fallible and that stresses can affect our ability to gather and process information, in turn leading to inaccurate mental models and lowered situation awareness [6]. Poor situation awareness can lead to errors that may compromise patient safety. It is therefore important that healthcare workers monitor their own well-being.

The aviation industry has developed the mnemonic IM SAFE as a self-assessment tool for individual workers to monitor themselves and to establish if they are safe to work [19]. The self-assessment mnemonic stands for:

- I – illness
- M – medication
- S – stress
- A – alcohol
- F – fatigue
- E – emotion.

Another strategy for self-monitoring is based on James Reason's 'three bucket method' [33] and the NHS Foresight training package [21]. The three bucket method was developed by Reason [13, 23] as a way to provide 'error wisdom' – that is, to help individuals to recognise situations where they are more likely to make errors. The aim is to increase individual mindfulness of those factors that may affect processing of information and performance of tasks. While not specifically developed as such, the method can be used by individuals to make an assessment of their individual stressors, the context and the tasks that may adversely affect them at that particular time in maintaining situation awareness.

The technique involves the individual asking themselves three questions:

1. *How safely are they able to work?*
   In answering this they need to consider such things as their level of knowledge, skill, experience and expertise. As well, they should evaluate their personal experiences such as fatigue, life events or illness to assess if these may potentially affect their capacity to undertake the tasks required.
2. *What is the current working environment like?*
   In answering this they need to consider such things as the physical environment and workspace, the workload, the resources (both human and material available), the equipment to be used, and the team management and organisation supports available.
3. *How error prone is the required task(s) or duties?*
   In answering this they need to consider the complexity or novelty of the task, the potential errors that could occur and the processes and procedures that need to be followed.

In considering these, the person thinks of three buckets – a self, a context and a task bucket (see Figure 7.2). As they consider each of the three questions they add to the bucket if there are negative factors associated with their assessment. The more that goes into each bucket, the more likely there are factors that may increase the likelihood of an incorrect decision or action. It is important to note that this is an indicator, not an absolute certainty, but it does provide the individual with a method of assessing their potential individual capacity to achieve and maintain situation awareness and avoid making errors. Full buckets do not mean it is certain that an error will occur, and empty buckets do not provide certainty that an error will not occur. However, undertaking this self-assessment at least raises the consciousness of individuals to those situation and human factors that increase the likelihood of error and can contribute to a loss of situation awareness.

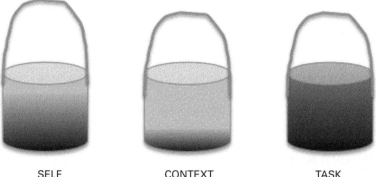

SELF　　　　　　　CONTEXT　　　　　　　TASK

Figure 7.2 Three bucket self-assessment tool to help individuals recognise the impact of individual stress factors that may increase the likelihood of error and a loss of situation awareness. Reproduced from *Beyond the Organisational Accident* by J. Reason in BMJ Quality and Safety in Healthcare v13 suppl 2 © 2004 with permission from BMJ Publishing Group Ltd

---

Exercise 7.3

Aim of the exercise: To practise assessment of individual capacity to maintain situational awareness.

What to do:

1. Think about a difficult shift you have had in the past. Now think of the three buckets of self, context and task and make an assessment of each of the factors that were present for you at the time.
2. How full were your buckets? Write a short list of key issues for each bucket.
3. Did you feel that your capacity to maintain situational awareness was satisfactory or did you think this might be compromised?
4. Discuss your answers with colleagues.

Summary

In this chapter we have discussed the role of situation awareness in maintaining patient safety. We identified the impact of cognitive, individual, context and task factors on an individual's facility to achieve and maintain situation awareness. Strategies that can be used to support the development of situation awareness were presented.

In the final chapter we will focus on goals for the future in the area of patient safety and the role of individual health practitioners in championing the lessons learnt so far. We will discuss briefly the principles of change management and how individuals can implement patient safety principles in their workplace. Finally, we will present a list of resources available for learning more about patient safety concepts.

The themes of this chapter relate to the WHO curriculum guideline topics of [19]:

- Why human factors are important to patient safety
- Being an effective team player.

The Exercise Feedback below provides an overview of the key points of this chapter.

EXERCISE FEEDBACK

Exercise 7.3 is a reflective exercise and as such there is no specific feedback for it.

Exercise 7.1

In this scenario the junior doctor is most likely basing her mental model on the academic knowledge that she has acquired during training that emphasises the relationship between alcohol abuse and poor parenting. She may also have had previous clinical experiences of cases where she has provided care to children when they have been injured as a direct or indirect result of their parents' alcohol abuse. Combining this knowledge and experience with the data she is cognitively processing about Tara which indicates she has been drinking heavily (smells strongly of alcohol, may be slurring words and emotionally disinhibited) will all lead Beverly to assume that Tara may be an alcoholic with poor parenting.

It is likely that if Tara was not displaying any signs or symptoms of high alcohol intake then Beverly would have formed a different mental model, one where she notes an unfortunate accident that can happen even when parents are vigilant.

Exercise 7.2

The PICU physician who gave the medication order was most likely working on a flawed mental model where he assumed the experience and knowledge of the team members and that the clinician receiving the order would know that the drugs in this situation are drawn up ready but are not given until everything is prepared and ready for the intubation to commence. He thus did not give any timing of the medication or instruction that it was to be drawn up but not given until later.

The nurse who gave the drug was most likely working on a mental model based either from previous experiences of other emergency situations or from her academic knowledge about emergency situations that when the order was given for a drug it was to be given immediately.

The accurate mental model that led to the correct actions by the team to remedy the situation was likely based on the team's clinical experience and knowledge. Noting that the child had suddenly desaturated they would have been cognitively searching for reasons why this happened – they may have consciously or unconsciously noted that the nurse was giving or had recently given medication (the nurse may have had the syringe in her hand or be standing next to the IV infusion, or she may have stated that the medication was given as ordered). They were able to link the two events and come up with an accurate mental model of the situation.

The following factors may have impacted on the situation for the nurse:

- **Cognitive factors:** From a cognitive perspective the nurse likely made an assumed connection where two pieces of confirmatory evidence appear, which can lead to inaccurate processing of the information and the wrong decision about actions to be taken. In this case it was an emergency situation and the physician had ordered emergency medication therefore the nurse made the decision that it needed to be given immediately.
- **Context factors:** The context was unfamiliar for the nurse as well as an emergency, time critical situation involving a child. All of these will have increased the stress levels for the nurse, which impedes effective cognitive functioning.
- **Individual factors:** The nurse may have been experiencing personal issues such as anxiety, fatigue, negative life events, stress or illness. As well, the nurse was in a new clinical environment, where she was inexperienced in both skills and knowledge.

- **Task factors:** The nurse was unfamiliar with the steps in the process for an emergent intubation – in this unit the process involved preparing but not giving the medication until the intubation tray was ready.

References

1. Wilson, K.A., et al., *Errors in the heat of battle: Taking a closer look at shared cognition breakdowns through teamwork.* Human Factors: The Journal of the Human Factors and Ergonomics Society, 2007. **49**(2): 243–256.
2. Woods, D., et al., *Behind Human Error,* 2010, Farnham, Surrey: Ashgate Publishing.
3. Reynard, J., J. Reynolds, and P. Stevenson, *Practical Patient Safety,* 2009, Oxford: Oxford University Press.
4. Endsley, M., *Theoretical underpinnings of situation awareness: A critical review,* in *Situation Awareness Analysis and Measurement,* M. Endsley and D. Garland, eds. 2000, Mahwah, NJ: Lawrence Erlbaum Associates.
5. Wright, S. and M. Fallacaro, *Predictors of situation awareness in student registered nurse anaesthetists.* AANA Journal, 2011. **79**(6): 484–490.
6. Dekker, S., *A Field Guide to Understanding Human Error,* 2006, Farnham, Surrey: Ashgate Publishing.
7. Salas, E., N. Cooke, and M. Rosen, *On teams, teamwork, and team performance: Discoveries and developments.* Human Factors, 2008. **50**(3): 540–547.
8. Endsley, M. *Situation models: An avenue to the modeling of mental models,* in *Proceedings of the Human Factors Ergonomics Society Annual Meeting,* 2000.
9. Dekker, S., *Patient Safety: A human factors approach,* 2011, Boca Raton, Florida: CRC Press.
10. *ISMP Medication Safety Alert! RG Inattentional blindness: what captures your attention? ... Reprinted with permission from ISMP Medication Safety Alert! Nurse Advise-ERR (ISSN 1550-6304) August 2009 Volume 7 Issue 8 Copyright 2009 Institute for Safe Medication Practices (ISMP).* Alberta RN, 2009. **65**(8): 16–17.
11. Wright, M., J. Taekman, and M. Endsley, *Objective measures of situation awareness in a simulated medical environment.* Quality and Safety in Health Care, 2004. **13**: i65–i71.
12. Toft, B. and H. Mascie-Taylor, *Involuntary automaticity: A work-system induced risk to safe health care.* Health Services Management Research, 2005. **18**: 211–216.
13. Reason, J., *Human error: Models and management.* BMJ, 2000. **320**: 768–770.
14. Endsley, M., *Situation awareness,* in *Human Factors and Ergonomics,* G. Salvendy, ed. 2012, New Jersey: John Wiley & Sons.
15. Baker, P., R. Day, and E. Salas, *Teamwork as an essential component of high-reliability organizations. (Public Policy and Research Agenda).* Health Services Research, 2006. **41**(4): 1576–1598.
16. Wachter, R., *Understanding Patient Safety.* 2nd ed. 2012, San Francisco: McGraw-Hill.

17. *The case of Elaine Bromiley* [accessed 26 April 2013]. Available from: www.chfg.org/wp-content/uploads/2012/02/ElaineBromileyAnonymous Report.pdf.
18. White, N., *Understanding the role of non-technical skills in patient safety.* Nursing Standard, 2012. **26**(26): 43–48.
19. *WHO Patient Safety Curriculum Guide: Multi-professional edition*, 2011, Geneva: World Health Organization.
20. Dekker, S., *Drift into Failure: From hunting broken components to understanding complex systems*, 2011, Farnham, Surrey: Ashgate Publishing.
21. Boakes, E., *Using foresight in safe nursing care.* Journal of Nursing Management, 2009. **17**: 212–217.
22. Proctor, R. and T. Van Zandt, *Human Factors in Simple and Complex Systems*, 2008, Boca Raton, Florida: CRC Press.
23. Reason, J., *The Human Contribution: Unsafe acts, accidents and heroic recoveries*, 2008, Farnham, Surrey: Ashgate Publishing.
24. Harrison, T., et al., *Use of cognitive aids in a simulated anesthetic crisis.* Anesthesia and Analgesia, 2006. **103**(3): 551–556.
25. Miller, K., W. Riley, and S. Davis, *Identifying key nursing and team behaviours to achieve high reliability.* Journal of Nursing Management, 2009. **17**: 247–255.
26. Degani, A. and E. Wiener, *Human Factors of Flight Deck Check Lists: The normal check-list.* Contract Report NCCC2-3771990, California: NASA Ames Research Center.
27. Thomassen, O., et al., *Implementation of checklists in healthcare: Learning from high reliability organisations.* Scandinavian Journal of Trauma, Resuscitation and Emergency Medicine, 2011. **19**: 53.
28. Reason, J., *Combating omission errors through task analysis and good reminders.* Quality and Safety in Health Care, 2002. **11**: 40–44.
29. Gaba , D., *The future vision of simulation in health care.* Quality and Safety in Health Care, 2004. **13**(Suppl. 1).
30. Youngberg, B., ed. *Patient Safety Handbook.* 2nd ed. 2013, Maryland: Jones & Bartlett Learning.
31. Gaba, D., *Have we gone too far in translating ideas from aviation to patient safety? No.* BMJ, 2011. **342**: c7310.
32. Yule, S., *Assessing intraoperative teamwork skills at the individual level: From research to implementation.* Proceedings of the Human Factors and Ergonomics Society Annual Meeting, 2012. **56**(1): 836–839.
33. Reason, J., *Beyond the organisational accident: The need for "error wisdom" on the frontline.* Quality and Safety in Health Care, 2004. **13**: 28–33.

8

Where To From Here?

Introduction

There have been considerable advances in the treatment and management of diseases over the last few centuries. However, while patients are benefiting from the knowledge of disease processes and the advances in technology that provide better diagnostic and treatment modalities, there is no doubt that being a recipient of care within the healthcare system is more risky than it should be for patients. There is still a lot of work required to make healthcare safe for patients [1].

In this final chapter we will focus on what the evidence suggests the future of the patient safety movement should be. We will also provide a template that can be used to record resources for future reference. There will be some discussion about change management theories and the barriers to implementing change. Finally, we will draw the chapter to a conclusion by discussing quality improvement tools and the role of individual health practitioners in championing the lessons learnt so far.

The Changing Landscape of Patient Safety in Healthcare

In previous chapters we presented the statistics for the incidence of adverse events in hospitals: some 1 in 10 patients will experience an adverse event, of these 1 in 5 will suffer a serious injury from the adverse event and 1 in 30 will die [2, 3]. Although these statistics relate to hospitalised patients, there is evidence that many patients in the community also suffer from errors related to the care they receive [4]. While these figures are based on research for developed countries, there is limited research for developing countries indicating that the risk for patients of suffering a serious adverse event is as high, if not higher, than in developed ones [4]. The need then for understanding, monitoring and managing the problem in both developed and developing countries is imperative. Before we move to a discussion of future goals it is important to recognise that there have been considerable advances in patient safety already. These advances provide a very solid platform for the future and highlight the significant developments that are possible across a relatively short timeframe.

Before the mid to late 1990s patient safety was not systematically recognised as a problem in the delivery of healthcare [5, 6]. In general the public came to know about major errors via the media – what normally followed was the search for someone to blame, and then the world moved on. Within healthcare, errors were either swept under the carpet or someone was identified as accountable and/or responsible and was dealt with either by retraining or sanction. Errors were perceived as rare and resulting from carelessness or incompetence [7]. However, following the IOM report [2] in 2000 along with various other studies in different countries which demonstrated the rates of errors in healthcare, the focus on patient safety increased. Further advances in access to information via the internet, together with heightened consumer awareness and expectations, have been added stimuli for a focus on patient safety. This increased focus has resulted in many positive steps to enhance patient safety.

Most importantly, patient safety is part of conversations not only within international, national and local political and health policy circles [1, 8–10], but also within health management and professional arenas. Patient safety is now the focus of research and systems improvement, and whether or not people agree with all the concepts surrounding it, there is now a general acceptance that there is a problem which needs attention. When an error occurs the response is changing from blaming and shaming individuals to a realisation that to recognise and prevent errors requires knowledge of the system and human factors that form part of the error chain. Contributing to this change has been an increase in the scope and quantum of research on patient safety that is now being carried out [1].

Many countries have identified that patient safety is a priority and have introduced various initiative. These include:

- centres for research into patient safety
- standards for credentialing and defining the scope of practice for medical practitioners
- medication safety initiatives
- surgical protocols such as 'correct patient, correct site, correct procedure'

- education of consumers to encourage involvement in monitoring healthcare delivered to them as individuals.

In addition, numerous countries have peak advisory groups charged with monitoring clinical governance within the health sector of their jurisdiction. Most have a requirement that certain sentinel events are reported to this committee. Patient adverse event reporting systems are now common within many healthcare organisations, with many required to report this information to national health bodies as well as taking part in accreditation programmes involving development of patient safety systems within the agency [1, 10–17].

Improved understanding about practical strategies that health professionals could adopt has been recognised as an important tactic to change behaviour at the 'sharp' end of care. With this in mind, as mentioned in the Introduction, the World Health Organization (WHO) recently developed a curriculum guide, with educational resources that can be used in undergraduate and postgraduate programmes for all health professionals [1]. The curriculum guide covers 11 topics considered essential knowledge for health practitioners. This book has been informed by the curriculum topics (see Table 0.1 for relationship to the WHO curriculum). However, despite the heightened awareness of the safety agenda, Lander and colleagues noted a serious shortage of educational programmes for clinical staff seeking to develop skills in enhancing safety in care settings [18].

In spite of the recent significant advances there is still a major problem with patient safety [1, 14]. It would seem that the more we understand about it, the more we recognise some of its complex characteristics and consequently how we might develop more sophisticated solutions. Significant research to gain an increased understanding about the structural and process factors that lead to errors remains a high priority. The need to target areas of recognised risk with evidence based interventions should also remain a priority for policy makers, funders, health organisations and individual practitioners [4, 19]. Organisations also need to be aware of how risks are communicated to different audiences and that there are many strategies and techniques that can be used effectively [20].

Thus the last two decades have witnessed important developments in patient safety but much work remains to be done. The need to change at both individual and organisational levels lies at the heart of future developments. At the same time it is clear that the safety agenda needs to be addressed across all facets of healthcare, and the responsibility for this lies at the feet of regulators, organisations and individuals.

Developing Through Change

We have covered many of the key areas that are vulnerable to errors in the chapters of this book. However, we have not yet discussed the strategies that need to be considered when thinking about implementing change. Change is a critical element in anything we do to develop solutions in these areas. Sometimes the change need will impact on everyone in the system and sometimes it may require a very personal commitment to working in a new way while recognising that many people don't like change. The next section will tackle this topic, as well as looking at the barriers to be contemplated when implementing change. Firstly, however, the following activity will provide you with some practice in accessing information about patient safety priorities.

Exercise 8.1

Aim of the exercise: To identify the different resources available to support you or your organisation change behaviour to implement patient safety initiatives.

What to do:

1. Spend some time accessing and reviewing the websites listed in Table 8.1. As you review each one complete the table by identifying the most recent research available on the website, the tools and resources that are available for you to access, as well as publications and other links that you can access from the websites. Feel free to add more resources that you find as you explore websites, books and publications. Keep this list and update it as you come across more information in your workplace or as you do further reading or study.
2. Consider the following questions:

    a. Who are these resources aimed at primarily?
    b. Who should they be aimed at?
    c. How realistic is it to think these could be used routinely?
    d. How might people at work respond to these?
    e. How could these responses be addressed?

3. Discuss and compare your findings with colleagues – you may want to add more information to your table following these discussions.

Table 8.1 Linking website information with resources available to support patient safety initiatives

Website	Patient involvement	Medication safety	Healthcare acquired infections	Teamwork and communication	Error reporting	Situation awareness	Human factors	Other links	Other information
Health & Disability Commissioner, New Zealand: www.hdc.org.nz									
World Health Organization 1: www.who.int/patientsafety/en/									
Agency for Healthcare Research and Quality, USA: www.ahrq.gov/qual/patientsafetyix.htm									
Institute for Healthcare Improvement, USA: www.ihi.org/knowledge/Pages/default.aspx									
Australian Commission on Safety and Quality in Health Care: www.safetyandquality.gov.au/ National Patient Safety Agency, National Health Service, UK: www.npsa.nhs.uk/									
Australian Institute of Health Innovation, Centre for Clinical Governance Research: www.aihi.unsw.edu.au/ccgr/									
World Health Organization 2: www.who.int/patientsafety/patients_for_patient/en/									

Change Management

In each chapter of this book we have identified different areas of safety where changes need to be made. However, so far, we have not addressed the change process itself. There are many change management theories. For example, incremental change management theories focus on small or minor changes within an organisation. Transitional change theories are useful when the aim is to move an organisation to a different structure or focus. Transformational change management theories are useful when the goal is to move to a whole new set of attitudes or methods. However, there are commonalities in all these theories which involve identifying the need for change, acknowledging the requirement for planning and implementing change and then ensuring there is a mechanism to monitor the sustainability of the changed practice [21–24].

Kurt Lewin's theory of change [25] has the elements described above. Even though it was developed in the 1940s it is still considered contemporary, and continues to be used extensively to provide understanding of the change process as well as a model on which planning to introduce change is based [21, 23]. In formulating his theory of change, Lewin maintained that individuals and groups strive to maintain the status quo and resist change. The forces that can change the status quo are driving forces (push towards or support change) or restraining forces (pull away from or restrain change). To bring about change, either the driving forces must be increased or the restraining forces decreased, or a combination of both (see Figure 8.1).

Lewin noted, however, that increasing the driving forces is not without cost. This is because any increase in driving forces generally impacts on group tensions. Increasing group tensions results in higher group fatigue, aggressiveness, emotion, and lower constructiveness. If this tension is increased beyond a certain point the group becomes dysfunctional. Lewin asserts that to achieve a desired change state, it is better to diminish the restraining forces rather than just increasing the driving ones [25]. Further to this, Lewin also identified that the forces that drive or resist change have the added characteristics of being either induced or owned. Induced forces are those imposed on the group or individual and are more likely to be resisted by the group. Those forces that are owned by the group, on the other hand, are more likely to be embraced and thus are more likely to overcome barriers to change.

Lewin's model describes change as a three-stage process – unfreezing, moving and refreezing. Lewin described the unfreezing stage as

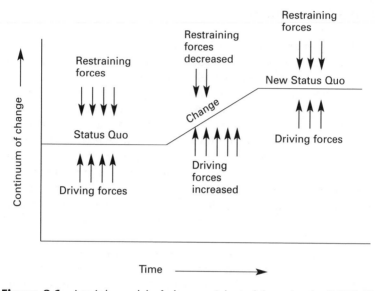

Figure 8.1   Lewin's model of change. Adapted from Lewin (1951) [25: 216]

'break(ing) open the shell of complacency and self-righteousness' and that to do this it 'is sometimes necessary to bring about deliberately an emotional stir up' [25: 330]. The unfreezing stage requires that the restraining and driving forces are identified and understood within the context that the change is to take place. There are two parts to unfreezing: the first is demonstrating the need for change in a way that convinces the participants to change their views or norms of current practice, and the second is ensuring the climate is one in which participants feel safe to embrace change [25, 26].

The second stage of the model is moving. This involves either increasing the driving forces or decreasing the restraining forces and comprises the processes of moving the group involved to the new changed state by carrying out the desired change in processes or behaviours. This may involve training and education for the new behaviours and/or planning and designing new work processes.

The final stage in Lewin's model is described as refreezing. This component requires rebalancing the driving and restraining forces. This can be achieved by a change in the group's goals, standards and values, and in the way a group sees itself and other groups within the social field. It may involve putting in place systems to reinforce the changed behaviour such as new ways to measure performance or organisational structural changes.

Although we may be familiar with change management theory, in reality there are many attempts to introduce changes to practice to improve patient safety which are never accepted or implemented as intended [27, 28]. In some instances changes are implemented successfully but are not sustained, and after the passing of time practices revert back to those that were in place before the change was introduced [28, 29]. These changes to practice fail not because the practice being changed is itself flawed, but rather because the processes used to introduce the change are defective or lack some essential elements needed to facilitate a successful, permanent change [30]. To maximise the likelihood of successful change implementation it is important to understand not only the elements that support the process but also the barriers that impede it. In the next section we will consider some of the barriers to change in healthcare, but first complete the following exercise.

Exercise 8.2

Aim of the exercise: To identify the facilitators and barriers to change.

What to do:

1. Consider the following scenario:

   Sean worked in a busy peri-operative unit. The workload was heavy and hours could be long. Recently the theatre manager introduced the 'surgical safety checklist', designed by WHO to decrease wrong patient/wrong surgery/wrong site occurrences. The majority of staff on the floor (including Sean) failed to understand the need for this change, perceiving that it was imposed on them by management without consultation, and that it was a waste of time, so they did everything they could to block it and avoid using it. After all, they knew that their record was 100 per cent on patient safety and they always checked patient consents closely and always got it right.

   One day, in an orthopaedic list the next patient, who was to have a total knee replacement, was brought into the theatre. The staff followed the usual routine (checking consent/checking marked limb) but didn't use the surgical safety checklist as was required. The patient was anaesthetised, prepped and then draped with the limb to be operated on exposed ready for the surgical procedure.

   The surgeon was just about to make the first incision when he stopped. 'Have we got the correct leg here, something is not right,' he queried. He got the staff to check his own notes; sure enough the consent was wrong and the wrong knee had been marked. The surgical team were about to

> *operate on the incorrect limb. In debriefing later they acknowledged that if they had used the surgical safety checklist they would most likely have picked this up as this requires the patient to confirm the operative area, and the surgeon to confirm verbally the site and the surgery. After that near miss, the surgical safety checklist was more widely appreciated within the theatre unit and incorporated into routine practice.*
>
> 2. Identify the driving and restraining forces before and after the near-miss event.
> 3. Write a list of strategies that could have been employed to gain acceptance of the WHO surgical safety list before the near-miss event.
> 4. Discuss your findings with colleagues and friends. What elements of what you have learnt can you apply in the future when you are involved in a change process designed to enhance safety?
> 5. Compare your findings with the Exercise Feedback section at the end of the chapter.

The Challenges of Change Management in Healthcare

There has been significant research into change processes in the health industry, and a number of common threads have been identified as key if a change management project is to succeed. Some of these are generic, applying to all change processes, and others are particular to those changes targeting patient safety. These common threads include:

- positive attitudes and values about patient safety and quality throughout the organisation
- organisational processes and systems that support safety and quality
- leadership and support from the leadership team
- key and influential clinician support and championing of the change
- team-based problem solving
- focus on positive patient outcomes
- involvement of patients in the care planning process
- data that supports the need for change
- those involved in the change have to be convinced of the need for change so there is ownership of the process

- change implementation process well resourced financially, and administratively
- a clear and logical plan for change [28, 30–33].

Of course these elements can all be present to varying degrees and change implementation can still fail. Within any organisation it is likely that groups and individuals may resist change. This can be for a variety of reasons including the barriers of organisational inertia, threats to group or individual expertise or power relationships, and fear of the unknown [23]. Health organisations are no different to any other organisation in terms of these barriers, but the context of health delivery does provide a unique aspect to them. These barriers fall into two categories: professional culture and organisational culture.

The health professional culture, which we have discussed previously in relation to communication difficulties and teamwork, can also act as a barrier to change. The authority and autonomous practice that is the dominant medical culture, and is also present to a lesser extent in the other health professions, can act as a significant change barrier. Occupying this influential position means that the beliefs and attitudes this group have about the process of care, and the systems underlying it, are pivotal to how the care is then delivered. These beliefs and attitudes are influenced by an education and training which emphasises that doctors need to be self-reliant, independent, autonomous and accountable to their profession [34].

Importantly, these early beliefs are often reinforced in the socialisation which young doctors receive as they enter practice – from those already in the medical profession as well as from other health professionals and the community who, by their own patterned reactions and interactions, reinforce the concept of medical dominance [35]. Finally, these attitudes and beliefs are maintained by what is described by McPherson and colleagues as the homophily principle [36]. This is the phenomenon where people tend to associate with others similar to themselves in terms of social situation, education, gender and race.

West et al. [37] assert that this phenomenon is strong in the medical profession, with the result that, as professionals, doctors have little contact with differing views. Because of this, doctors are less likely to be exposed to new or differing information from outside their medical professional circles, and remain unaware of changed trends or expectations that do not impinge immediately on their sphere of practice. This, combined with the medical profession's position of power within health organisations, means that if this group do not see a need for change then they can be extremely resistant to change initiatives [28, 38]. They can also help to shape the views of other professional groups in the system.

An organisational culture which is not supportive of patient safety acts as a major barrier to change. Healthcare is unique in that even when adverse incidents or even a major failure are made public, the customers (patients and families) continue to use the service. This is particularly so when the hospital or health service is the only one available in the community. Contrast this to a major airline failure or nuclear industry failure. In these situations, the customers can boycott the service, or if the risk is extreme, the organisation will be shut down until remedial action is put in place.

In health, while people continue to get sick and require healthcare, a hospital may be the focus of investigation but patients will still present for care [39]. Day-to-day care activity within the hospital does not change, and although patients and families may have a heightened anxiety about something going wrong, for most, their individual interactions with health professionals continue to be positive. This creates a different mindset and incentive for both direct care health professionals and health management when business continues as normal. Thus, for health organisations, the need to commit human and financial resources in an environment where these are scarce does not carry the same organisational imperative as it does for other industries, where failure to fix a problem may result in the organisation having to cease operating [39].

A positive patient safety culture within an organisation is essential to support change. Strong leadership and a commitment to patient safety, as well as the structures and processes that support it, are necessary ingredients to create a culture that embraces and welcomes change as an inevitable part of improving patient safety.

Unfortunately there is no 'magic' recipe that will ensure changes are implemented successfully and will be sustained. To implement change requires not only understanding of healthcare cultural behaviours and context barriers that can sabotage change efforts, but also an understanding of those strategies within the supportive context that are most likely to succeed in implementing change. Before attempting any change process a full assessment should be undertaken to identify the facilitators and barriers to change within the particular context. In many instances you yourself will not be in a position to instigate a major change process, but it is highly likely that you will be involved during your career in healthcare organisations with initiatives aimed at improving patient safety. 'Quality improvement' is a term many of you may be familiar with. It describes the processes used to improve systems and functions, and has been in use for decades in other industries. It is now becoming common in healthcare. We will discuss quality improvement in the next section, but before we do complete the following exercise.

Exercise 8.3

Aim of the exercise: Further work on identifying the facilitators and barriers to change.

What to do:

1. Think about a time you were involved in a change process that significantly altered the way things were done. This can be in your workplace, or maybe in the school where you are studying or in your personal life.
2. Write down what was changed and how it was changed.
3. Now identify if the change was successfully implemented. If so why, if not why not? What specific strategies were employed?
4. Who else was influential in the change process?
5. What were the primary motivations for the change?
6. Discuss your findings with colleagues and friends. What elements of what you have learnt can you apply in the future when you are involved in a change process?

Quality Improvement

Throughout this book we have looked at areas of risk for patient safety, as well as identifying strategies that can be used to mitigate these risks. Furthermore, in Chapter 6 we examined ways we could learn from errors using adverse event reporting systems, emphasising the importance of using this knowledge to improve patient safety. Quality improvement is concerned with utilising this information along with other indicators to improve care.

Essentially, quality improvement focuses on examining the way things are being done and then deciding if there is a better way to do them. There are several ways this can be done, including:

- using event reports from incident monitoring systems, incident investigations, professional journals and conferences, coroners' inquests, technical and therapeutic notifications and legal cases to identify areas of patient safety risk
- auditing current processes against the policy or procedure that details the requirements, identifying the deficits and then putting strategies in place to improve compliance with the policy or procedure
- measuring outcomes of certain procedures or practices against benchmarks and identifying where improvements can be made
- researching the latest evidence on a particular process, procedure or practice and then comparing this with how it is done in your particular organisation; if there are differences then taking steps to change the process, procedure or practice to reflect the latest evidence [33].

The principles that underpin successful quality improvement activities use our understanding of change management discussed above – that is, using the three stages of unfreezing, movement and freezing to apply our change process. Moreover, we need to ensure that the key elements of successful change management projects are present, and that we have identified the barriers that may derail the change process. There are several quality improvement tools that can be used, including Six Sigma, Total Quality Management, Lean, Business Process Redesign, and Plan, Do, Study, Act (PDSA) [40–44]. We will examine just one of these – the PDSA tool, which is the most common in healthcare [1]. Information about the other tools is available in the articles referenced.

The PDSA tool is a small scale, bottom-up approach to improvement [29]. Figure 8.2 illustrates the cycle. There are two parts to this method. The first asks the questions:

- What are we trying to achieve?
- How will we know that we have achieved it?
- What do we need to do to achieve the changes we want?

The second part involves putting the answers to the questions into action:

- Plan: plan the change to be implemented or tested
- Do: carry out the test or change
- Study: study the data before and after the change
- Act: act on the information and plan the next change cycle [29].

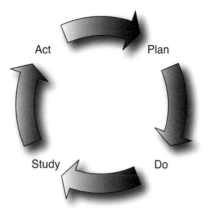

Figure 8.2 The Plan–Do–Study–Act cycle. Adapted from *WHO Patient Safety Curriculum Guide: Multi-professional edition* (2011) [1]

It is important to note that although the improvement activities are described in a linear fashion, this should actually be an ongoing cyclic process so that once strategies for improvement are instituted the process keeps on going until it is established that the improvement has been made and sustained.

The factors that will support success are similar to those detailed in our discussion about change management challenges above. The importance of these factors applied to quality improvement strategies cannot be emphasised enough, so we will take time here to reiterate those issues as they apply to quality improvement. The following issues need to be considered:

- The improvement team needs to involve those people who are or will be involved in the change being implemented. Include someone who is influential in the change context who will champion the change.
- The team needs to clearly articulate the objectives they are aiming to achieve. These need timeframes and a clear description of the desired outcomes.
- The team needs to define how they will measure achievement of the objectives.
- The team needs to identify the changes that are required to achieve the objectives they have set.
- The team then needs to undertake Plan, Do, Study, Act [45].

The implementation of changes and quality improvement activities to improve patient safety, in the main, requires teams of people. It is likely that you will have the opportunity to be involved in one of these teams in the future. However, until you are able to participate in a team project it is imperative that you seize all opportunities as an individual practitioner to improve patient safety. There are things that you as an individual in professional practice can do that support patient safety. We will discuss these in the next section.

What Can Individual Practitioners Do to Support Patient Safety?

The most important and effective thing you can do in your daily professional practice is to strive to achieve the highest standards of evidence based care. This should include the following strategies:

- Actively include patients and families in the planning and delivery of care that you give. Maintain continuity of care for patients by ensuring that you document care and communicate appropriately with other health professionals.
- Champion patient safety. It may not be easy in a complex multi-professional organisation and will depend to a large extent on the organisational culture, but remember – change happens from small beginnings.
- Seek opportunities to be involved in improvement activities, and ask and learn about tools and strategies to improve patient safety.
- Develop an awareness of the particular risks to patient safety in your ward, department, unit or community setting. Once you have identified these, implement into your daily practice evidence based practice protocols for the minimisation of errors. This could be as simple as ensuring that you follow hand hygiene principles on every occasion; or it may be that you work in an area where patients are at risk of falls or the development of pressure areas so you could introduce risk assessment protocols to manage these hazards. If you are involved in the prescription or administration of medication reviews, what are the particular issues that need to be addressed in this context? You have been introduced to some of the tools and resources in this book, but you will need to continually search for and put the most up to date evidence based practice in place.
- Be mindful and incorporate the principles of good communication. Utilise the tools of SBAR and CUS (see Chapter 6) – even if your

organisation has not formally adopted these they still provide an excellent tool for any individual practitioner to structure communication so it is clear and contains the required information.

• Be assertive in actively championing patient safety, but at the same time be aware of the importance of self-care.

• Identify the processes that are in place to report and manage adverse events in your workplace. Actively contribute to these processes.

• Finally, remember humans are fallible and they make mistakes. Regularly assess how error prone you may be in your work using the three bucket method discussed in the previous chapter. Review self, context and task for stressors that make it more likely that errors may happen. Identify contingencies to deal with the stressors to reduce the risk of errors.

Summary

Throughout the book we identified strategies for improving patient safety. However, knowing about these strategies is of little value if we do not understand how they can be implemented successfully in the organisational context. The focus of this chapter was to introduce the reader to the principles of change management and some of the main barriers to change. A general discussion about quality improvement followed, along with some discussion of the specific quality improvement tool Plan, Do, Study, Act (PDSA).

The strategies we have identified to enhance patient safety are much easier to achieve if you are working in an organisation that values and gives priority to patient safety. However, if this is not the case you can still make a difference as an individual. There may be times when this is difficult or you may be criticised for 'bucking' the norm, but small things make a difference so stay committed to these principles of patient safety and eventually you will be part of the tide of change. Such a commitment is not only in your own best interests – it is also a crucial element in the safekeeping of those we care for as health professionals.

EXERCISE FEEDBACK

Exercise 8.1 and 8.3 are reflective exercises and as such there is no specific feedback for these.

Exercise 8.2

In this scenario the drivers for change before the near-miss event included:

- the evidence that the surgical safety checklist has been shown to decrease adverse events
- the fact that the surgical safety checklist is designed using human factors principles that are less likely to result in automatic responses
- evidence that wrong site surgery – although rare – still occurs.

Other driving forces that may have been present but are not evident in this scenario description are:

- positive attitudes and values about patient safety and quality throughout the organisation
- organisational processes and systems that support safety and quality
- leadership and support from the leadership team.

The restraining forces against change before the near-miss event included:

- staff were not convinced about the rationale for change
- staff were not involved in the decision to change or the planning and subsequent implementation
- lack of key and influential clinician support to champion the change.

Other restraining forces that may have been present but are not evident in the scenario description are:

- health professional culture – authority and autonomy that is the dominant medical culture
- organisational culture that does not support change
- lack of patients' involvement in care processes
- lack of data to support change.

References

1. *WHO Patient Safety Curriculum Guide: Multi-professional edition*, 2011, Geneva: World Health Organization.
2. IOM, *To Err is Human: Building a safer health care system*, 2000, Washington, DC: National Academy Press.

3. Wilson, R., et al., *The quality in Australian health care study.* MJA, 1995. **193**: 458–471.
4. Jha, A., N. Prasopa-Plazier, and I. Larizgoitia, *Patient safety research: An overview of the global evidence.* Quality and Safety in Health Care, 2010. **19**: 42–47.
5. Leape, L., *Patient safety: What have we learned? Where are we going?* in *4th Australasian Conference on Safety and Quality in Health Care.* 2006. Melbourne, Australia.
6. Leape, L. and D. Berwick, *Five years after To Err is Human: What have we learnt?* JAMA, 2005. **293**: 2384–2390.
7. Wachter, R., *Understanding Patient Safety.* 2nd ed. 2012, San Francisco: McGraw-Hill.
8. *WHO Draft Guidelines for Adverse Event Reporting and Learning Systems.* 2005 [accessed 15 July 2008]. Available from: www.who.patient/safety.
9. *WHO Draft Guidelines for Adverse Event Reporting Systems and Learning Systems,* 2005, Geneva: World Health Organization.
10. *Summary of the Evidence on Patient Safety: Implications for research,* 2008, Geneva: World Alliance for Patient Safety, World Health Organization.
11. *Credentialing and Defining the Scope of Clinical Practice for the Medical Practitioners in Queensland,* 2009, Queensland Health.
12. Barraclough, B. and J. Birch, *Health care safety and quality: Where have we been and where are we going?* eMJA, 2006. **184**: s48–s40.
13. Braithwaite, J., et al., *Health service accreditation as a predictor of clinical and organisational performance: A blinded, random, stratified study.* Quality and Safety in Health Care, 2010. **19**(1): 14–21.
14. Dekker, S., *Patient Safety: A human factors approach,* 2011, Boca Raton, Florida: CRC Press.
15. Longo, D.R., et al. *The Long Road to Patient Safety: A status report on patient safety systems.* JAMA, 2005. **294**: 2858–2865.
16. Pronovost, P.J., M.R. Miller, and R.M. Wachter, *Tracking progress in patient safety: An elusive target.* JAMA, 2006. **296**: 696–699.
17. Wilson, R. and M. Van der Weyden, *The safety of Australian healthcare: 10 years after QAHCS.* eMJA, 2005. **182**: 260–261.
18. Lander, J., et al., *Learning about quality and safety in an on-line learning environment.* Focus on Health Professional Education: A Multi-Disciplinary Journal, 2010. **12**(1): 31–38.
19. Jha, A., ed. *Summary of the Evidence on Patient Safety: Implications for research.* 2008, Geneva: WHO Press.
20. Lundgren, R. and A. McMakin, *Risk Communication: A handbook for communicating environmental, safety and health risk,* 2009, Hoboken, N: John Wiley & Sons.
21. Burke, W., *Organization change: Theory and practice.* 2nd ed. 2008, Thousand Oaks, California: Sage Publications.
22. Ellis, J. and C. Hartley, *Managing and Coordinating Nursing Care.* 5th ed. 2009, Philadelphia: Lippincott Williams & Wilkins.
23. Robbins, S., B. Millett, and T. Waters-Marsh, *Organisational Behaviour.* 4th ed. 2004, Frenchs Forest: Pearson Education Australia.
24. Shortell, S. and A. Kaluzny, eds. *Health Care Management: Organization design and behavior.* 5th ed. 2006, Thomson Delmar Learning: New York.

25. Lewin, K., *Frontiers in group dynamics*, in *Field Theory in Social Science*, D. Cartwright, ed. 1951, Harper & Brothers: New York: 188–238.
26. Schein, E., *Organizational Culture and Leadership*, 1985, San Francisco: Jossey-Bass.
27. Hurley, C., F. Baum, and H. van Eyk, *Designing better health care in the South: A case study of unsuccessful transformational change in public sector health service reform.* Australian Journal of Public Administration, 2004. **82**(2): 31–41.
28. McGrath, K., et al., *Implementing and sustaining transformational change in health care: Lessons learnt about clinical process redesign.* eMJA, 2008. **188**: S32–S35.
29. Powell, A., R. Rushmer, and H. Davies, *Practitioner led rapid cycle change.* British Journal of Healthcare Management, 2009. **15**(5): 218–222.
30. Fitzgerald, L., et al., *Service improvement in healthcare: Understanding change capacity and change context.* Clinician in Management, 2007. **15**: 61–74.
31. Brazier, A. and B. Wren, *Organizational matters.* Clinical Child Psychology and Psychiatry, 2009. **14**: 475.
32. Gluyas, H., S. Alliex, and P. Morrison, *Do inquiries into health system failures lead to change in clinical governance systems?* Collegian, 2011. **18**(4): 147–156.
33. Wolff, A. and S. Taylor, *Enhancing Patient Safety: A practical guide to improving quality and safety in hospitals*, 2009, Sydney: MJA Books.
34. Stanton, P., *The politics of healthcare: Managing the healthcare workforce*, in *Managing Clinical Processes in Health Services*, R. Sorenson and R. Iedema, eds. 2008, Elsevier: Sydney: 35–49.
35. Allsop, J., *Medical dominance in a changing world: The UK case.* Health Sociology Review, 2006. **15**: 444–457.
36. McPherson, M., L. Smith-Lovin, and J. Cook, *Birds of a feather: Homophily in social networks.* Annual Review of Sociology, 2001. **27**: 415–444.
37. West, E., et al., *Hierarchies and cliques in the social networks of health care professionals: Implications for the design of dissemination strategies.* Social Science of Medicine, 1999. **48**: 633–646.
38. West, E., *Sociological contributions to patient safety*, in *Patient Safety: Research into practice*, K. Walshe and R. Boaden, eds. 2008, Maidenhead, Berkshire: Open University Press: 19–30.
39. Walshe, K. and S. Shortell, *When things go wrong: How health care organisations deal with major failures.* Health Affairs, 2004. **23**: 103–111.
40. Powell, A., R. Rushmer, and H. Davies, *Quality improvement TQM and CQI approaches.* British Journal of Healthcare Management, 2009. **15**(3): 114–120.
41. Powell, A., R. Rushmer, and H. Davies, *Effective quality improvement: BPR.* British Journal of Healthcare Management, 2009. **15**(4): 166–171.
42. Powell, A., R. Rushmer, and H. Davies, *Effective quality improvement: Lean.* British Journal of Healthcare Management, 2009. **15**(6): 270–275.
43. Powell, A., R. Rushmer, and H. Davies, *Effective quality improvement: Recognising the challenges.* British Journal of Healthcare Management, 2009. **15**(1): 17–21.
44. Powell, A., R. Rushmer, and H. Davies, *Effective quality improvement: Six Sigma.* British Journal of Healthcare Management, 2009. **15**(7): 322–326.
45. Powell, A., R. Rushmer, and H. Davies, *Effective quality improvement: Some necessary conditions.* British Journal of Healthcare Management, 2009. **15**(2): 62–68.

Index